The New Sjogren's Syndrome Handbook

EDITOR

DANIEL J. WALLACE, MD

ASSOCIATE EDITORS

Evelyn J. Bromet, PHD

Arthur Grayzel, MD

Katherine Morland Hammitt, MA

Stuart S. Kassan, MD

Frederick B. Vivino, MD

A publication of the SJOGREN'S SYNDROME FOUNDATION

The **New**
Sjogren's
Syndrome
Handbook

REVISED AND EXPANDED THIRD EDITION

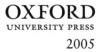

OXFORD
UNIVERSITY PRESS
2005

OXFORD

UNIVERSITY PRESS

Oxford   New York
Auckland   Bangkok   Buenos Aires   Cape Town   Chennai
Dar es Salaam   Delhi   Hong Kong   Istanbul   Karachi   Kolkata
Kuala Lumpur   Madrid   Melbourne   Mexico City   Mumbai   Nairobi
São Paulo   Shanghai   Taipei   Tokyo   Toronto

Copyright © 2005 by The Sjogren's Syndrome Foundation

Published by Oxford University Press, Inc.
198 Madison Avenue, New York, New York 10016
www.oup.com

Oxford is a registered trademark of Oxford University Press

Library of Congress Cataloging-in-Publication Data
The new Sjogren's syndrome handbook / editor, Daniel J. Wallace;
associate editors, Evelyn J. Bromet . . . [et al.]—3rd ed., rev. and expanded
p. cm.
"A publication of the Sjogren's Syndrome Foundation"
Includes bibliographical references and index
ISBN-13 978-0-19-517228-7
ISBN 0-19-517228-0
1. Sjogren's syndrome—Popular works.
I. Wallace, Daniel J. (Daniel Jeffrey), 1949–
II. Bromet, Evelyn J.
III. Sjogren's Syndrome Foundation.
RC 647.5.S5 N49 2005
616.7'75—dc22   2003027681

3 5 7 9 8 6 4

Printed in the United States of America
on acid-free paper

CONTENTS

PREFACE

SJOGREN'S SYNDROME is an autoimmune disorder that afflicts women and men of all ages, with perimenopausal women representing the highest-risk group. Because it is a disorder that can manifest itself in many different ways, Sjogren's syndrome may go undetected and undiagnosed for years, which in turn can lead to physical damage, disability, and emotional suffering. This was the situation facing Elaine Harris in 1983 when she founded the Sjogren's Syndrome Foundation (SSF). Mrs. Harris recognized that patients need to be knowledgeable about Sjogren's syndrome if they are to successfully navigate the medical care system to get the proper diagnosis and best possible treatment. Hence in 1989, she spearheaded the effort within the SSF to produce the first *Sjogren's Syndrome Handbook*. The first volume was soon followed by a second edition, *The New Sjogren's Syndrome Handbook*, edited by Steven Carsons, MD, and Elaine Harris, that took into account new insights from research about this complex, multifaceted disease.

This new book, edited by Dr. Daniel J. Wallace in collaboration with members of the foundation's medical and scientific advisory board, substantially expands and updates medical information on the causes and consequences of Sjogren's syndrome. The various chapters incorporate discoveries from recent cutting-edge investigations about the origins and treatments of Sjogren's syndrome. There are chapters on the various organ systems that can be affected, on possible psychological impacts, and on various treatment options, as well as an appendix enumerating the resources available for patients with the disease. The book also addresses the concerns of many patients with Sjogren's syndrome who also have other chronic health problems, such as rheumatoid arthritis, chronic fatigue syndrome, fibromyalgia, diabetes, high blood pressure, and osteoporosis. Thus, this book offers a comprehensive glimpse into the many faces of Sjogren's and the patterns and consequences of comorbid conditions.

It's no secret that if you don't ask the right questions, you won't get the right answers. This book is specifically intended to give patients a comprehensive vehicle from which to launch questions and evaluate answers.

Sjogren's patients are all too aware that the disorder encompasses more symptoms than just dry eyes and dry mouth. But many doctors and health care providers are not aware of all of its potential somatic sequelae. This book is thus intended to be a resource that patients can share with their doctor and other health care providers so that they have the most up-to-date information on diagnosis and treatment. And make sure that family and friends read this book as well, so that they too will better understand what their loved ones are experiencing from day to day.

For the SSF, this new *Handbook* has special significance because educating patients and their families about Sjogren's syndrome and increasing public and professional awareness are two of our primary missions. The SSF also has a third mission—that of promoting research into new treatments and a cure. As an epidemiologist and Sjogren's patient, I am optimistic that this new edition of the *Handbook* will stimulate clinical investigators by exposing them to the diverse manifestations of the disease and by increasing their awareness of its public health impact.

Lastly, I hope that this book will be read and studied by the general public, clinicians, psychologists, epidemiologists, and biomedical scientists worldwide. We all have to work together to develop effective interventions to alleviate or avert the symptoms and—sooner rather than later, I hope—to develop the means to prevent its occurrence.

Evelyn J. Bromet, PhD
Past chair, Sjogren's Syndrome Foundation Publications Committee
Professor of Psychiatry and Preventive Medicine
State University of New York, Stony Brook

CONTRIBUTORS

MIRHELEN MENDES ABREU, MD Rheumatology Discipline, Faculdade de Ciências Medicas, Universidade do Estado do Rio de Janeiro

JOAN E. BRODERICK, PhD Assistant Professor of Psychiatry and Behavioral Science, Program Director, Applied Behavioral Medical Research Institute, State University of New York, Stony Brook

EVELYN J. BROMET, PhD Professor of Psychiatry and Preventive Medicine, State University of New York, Stony Brook

STEVEN CARSONS, MD Chief, Division of Rheumatology, Allergy and Immunology, Winthrop University Hospital, Mineola, New York

AIKATERINI D. CHRYSOCHOU, MD Registrar in Rheumatology, Department of Pathophysiology, School of Medicine, National University of Athens

TROY E. DANIELS, DDS, MS Professor of Oral Medicine and Pathology, Schools of Dentistry and Medicine, University of California, San Francisco

REZA DANA, MD, MPH Associate Professor of Ophthalmology, Harvard University School of Medicine, Boston

PHILIP C. FOX, DDS President, P. C. Fox Consulting, LLC, and Visiting Scientist, Carolinas Medical Center, Charlotte, North Carolina

ROBERT I. FOX, MD, PhD Department of Rheumatology, Scripps Memorial Hospital and Research Foundation, La Jolla, California

ARTHUR GRAYZEL, MD, MACR Emeritus Professor of Medicine, New York University, and Past President, Sjogren's Syndrome Foundation

ABHA GULATI, MD Postdoctoral Research Fellow, Harvard University School of Medicine, Boston

DAVID S. HALLEGUA, MD Clinical Instructor, Cedars-Sinai/UCLA School of Medicine, Los Angeles

KATHERINE MORLAND HAMMITT, MA Director of Research Development and Public Policy, Sjogren's Syndrome Foundation, Bethesda, Maryland

JOHN HARLEY, MD Professor of Medicine, University of Oklahoma College of Medicine, Oklahoma City

LAMA HASHISH, MD Fellow in Rheumatology, University of Oklahoma Health Sciences Center, Oklahoma City

STUART S. KASSAN, MD, FACP, FACR Clinical Professor of Medicine, University of Colorado Health Sciences Center, Denver

ROBERT S. LEBOVICS, MD, FACS Head and Neck Surgical Group, New York, and Surgical Consultant, National Institutes of Health, Bethesda, Maryland

MICHAEL A. LEMP, MD Clinical Professor of Ophthalmology, Georgetown and George Washington University Schools of Medicine, Washington, DC

ROGER ABRAMINO LEVY, MD Rheumatology Discipline, Faculdade de Ciências Medicas, Universidade do Estado do Rio de Janeiro

CLIO P. MAVRAGANI, MD Fellow in Rheumatology, Department of Pathophysiology, School of Medicine, National University of Athens

JEANNE L. MELVIN, MS, OTR/L, FAOTA Past Program Manager, Fibromyalgia and Chronic Pain Program, Cedars-Sinai Medical Center, Los Angeles; Private Practice, Beverly Hills, California

SERENA MORRISON, MD National Eye Institute, National Institutes of Health, Bethesda, Maryland

HARALAMPOS M. MOUTSOPOULOS, MD, FACP, FRCP (Edin) Professor and Chairman, Department of Pathophysiology, School of Medicine, National University of Athens

STANLEY R. PILLEMER, MD Sjogren's Syndrome Clinic, Gene Therapy and Therapeutics Branch, National Institute of Dental and Craniofacial Research, National Institutes of Health, Bethesda, Maryland

AMR SAWALHA, MD Rheumatology Fellow, University of Michigan, Ann Arbor

JANINE SMITH, MD Deputy Clinical Director, National Eye Institute, National Institutes of Health, Bethesda, Maryland

FOTINI C. SOLIOTIS, MD, MRCP (UK) Specialist Registrar in Rheumatology, Royal Free Hospital, London, and Visiting Rheumatology Fellow,

Department of Pathophysiology, School of Medicine, National University of Athens

NEHAD R. SOLOMAN, MD Rheumatology Fellow, Winthrop University Hospital—Nassau University Medical Center, Mineola, New York

MARILYN A. SOLSKY, MD Attending Physician, Cedars-Sinai Medical Center, Los Angeles

HARRY SPIERA, MD Clinical Professor of Medicine, Mount Sinai School of Medicine, New York

ROBERT F. SPIERA, MD Associate Clinical Professor of Medicine, Albert Einstein College of Medicine, Director of Rheumatology, Beth Israel Medical Center, New York

NORMAN TALAL, MD Adjunct Professor of Medicine, New York University School of Medicine

SWAMY VENUTURUPALLI, MD Clinical Instructor, Cedars-Sinai Medical Center, David Geffen School of Medicine at the University of California, Los Angeles

VERONICA SILVA VILELA, MD Rheumatology Discipline, Faculdade de Ciências Medicas, Universidade do Estado do Rio de Janeiro

FREDERICK B. VIVINO, MD, FACR Chief, Division of Rheumatology, University of Pennsylvania Medical Center—Presbyterian, Penn Sjogren's Syndrome Center, Philadelphia

DANIEL J. WALLACE, MD Clinical Professor of Medicine, Cedars-Sinai Medical Center, David Geffen School of Medicine at the University of California, Los Angeles

MICHAEL H. WEISMAN, MD Director, Division of Rheumatology, Cedars-Sinai Medical Center, David Geffen School of Medicine at the University of California, Los Angeles

AVA J. WU, DDS Associate Clinical Professor of Oral Medicine, University of California, San Francisco School of Dentistry

Introduction: Why Write a Book on Sjogren's Syndrome?

ONE AMERICAN IN 70 has a mysterious eponymous condition known as Sjogren's syndrome. Named after a Swedish ophthalmologist who described its salient features 70 years ago, until recently Sjogren's resided in a nosologic purgatory, with its manifestations misunderstood, underappreciated, and ignored. An international consensus has finally been derived regarding what the term *Sjogren's* refers to. Now that organized science has finally come to terms (literally) with this syndrome, a number of insights elucidated by Sjogrenologists has been rapidly forthcoming. The collective wisdom of these investigators has recently resulted in the publication of prescient findings that serve to emphasize the importance of research into this area and will have implications far beyond the syndrome itself. The Sjogren's Syndrome Foundation has endeavored to collect the most relevant facts relating to the condition and publish them in this handbook. It is our hope that researchers, clinicians, physicians, allied health professionals, and dentists, as well as patients and their families, will be able to use this resource.

Why should we write a book on Sjogren's? Sjogren's is an autoimmune condition that affects the whole body, especially musculoskeletal and glandular tissues. It can exist as a primary condition or be a concomitant feature of rheumatoid arthritis, systemic lupus erythematosus, scleroderma, or other rheumatic disorders. According to the National Institutes of Health, between 14 million and 22 million Americans have an autoimmune condition, and 120 such conditions have been identified to date. Approximately 20 percent of this group have Sjogren's syndrome. Sjogren's is perceived incorrectly as being rare and does not receive a strong focus in medical education. Its symptoms are subtle and can be intermittent or nonspecific. It has been estimated that symptoms are present for a mean of six years before it is properly diagnosed. This is unfortunate, because a delayed diagnosis drastically alters quality of life. For example, up to 50 percent of individuals with Sjogren's report some degree of social isolation due to their symptoms, 62 percent have serious dental complications (e.g., caries), and 38 percent report significant musculoskeletal impairments. Most importantly, approximately 5–10 percent of those with primary Sjogren's develop a lymphoproliferative malignancy. Sjogren's is almost unique among autoimmune disorders in its ability to result in lymphoma in certain cases. This link could be exploited by researchers to help us understand many of the common immunologic features shared by cancer and autoimmune disorders.

Although Sjogren's is the second most common autoimmune condition affecting the musculoskeletal system, it ranks eighth in terms of research funding. Studies aimed at finding the cause of and cure for this syndrome will ultimately save taxpayers billions of dollars in lost wages and productivity, as well as improve lifestyle for many. We hope that our efforts will result in increased awareness and improved understanding of this underappreciated syndrome. This especially applies to patients, their families, and physicians and allied health professionals assisting in patient care.

This editor gratefully acknowledges the help of Katherine Hammitt, Director of Research and Public Policy for the Sjogren's Syndrome Foundation, for rounding up difficult-to-access statistics on the impact of the syndrome in the United States. The sources supporting this data are available from the national office upon request.

Daniel J. Wallace, MD
Clinical Professor of Medicine
Cedars-Sinai Medical Center
David Geffen School of Medicine at the
University of California, Los Angeles
November 2003

PART I

Introduction
and Definitions

The term *Sjogren's* does not tell the casual reader much about what the syndrome is. In this section, we will learn that although its features have been observed for hundreds of years, the first comprehensive description of the syndrome did not take place until 1933. The publication of statistically validatable criteria for Sjogren's has finally enabled investigators to not only define what it consists of but elucidate who develops the syndrome and how it is classified.

1 The History of Sjogren's Syndrome

THE FIRST CASE REPORT describing what we now know to be Sjogren's syndrome appeared in 1882, when the German physician Theodor Leber described filamentary keratitis (mucous strands that attach to and inflame the cornea). In 1888, surgeon Johann Mikulicz presented to the Society for Scientific Medicine at Königsberg the case of a 42-year-old East Prussian farmer with painless parotid, lacrimal, and submandibular gland swelling. The term *Mikulicz's syndrome* was commonly used to describe other conditions associated with parotid gland swelling, such as tuberculosis and lymphoma. Later that year, the London physician W. B. Hadden presented to the Clinical Society the case of a 65-year-old female with dry mouth and inability to tear whose condition responded to tincture of jaborandi (pilocarpine).

It took 30 more years for evidence of a "syndrome" to emerge. In 1926, Henri Gougerot in Paris described three patients with salivary gland enlargement and mucous membrane and vulvar atrophy and dryness. In 1927, Houwer connected filamentary keratitis with arthritis. And in 1933, the ophthalmologist Henrik Sjogren published his seminal monograph (not translated into English until 1943) in which he described a series of 19 patients with dry eye and dry mouth, of whom 13 also had arthritis. He coined the term *keratoconjunctivitis sicca* and used rose bengal staining to study the ocular surface for abnormalities due to dryness. Sjogren would go on to publish 15 more papers on the subject and practice ophthalmology; he retired in 1965 and died in 1986.

In 1953, William Morgan and Benjamin Castleman rediscovered and popularized Sjogren's work (which had received little attention) and elaborated upon its histopathologic features. Kurt Bloch and colleagues noted that Sjogren's could exist by itself or be secondary to other autoimmune disorders in 1955. In the 1950s and 1960s, Joseph Bunim, Norman Talal, and their students were instrumental in publishing the clinical presentation, natural history, and laboratory features of large numbers of Sjogren's patients and associating the syndrome with lymphoma. Even though Sjogren's antibodies (anti-Ro/SSA and anti-La/SSB) were discovered in the late 1960s, it took another 30 years for autoimmune Sjogren's to be differentiated from other causes of dry eye and dry mouth, such as HIV infection and hepatitis, in official classifications. This finally allowed clinical trials of medications for the treatment of Sjogren's syndrome to be undertaken.

2 What Is Sjogren's Syndrome?

IN THIS CHAPTER Sjogren's syndrome will be described and classified by means of its signs, symptoms, autoimmune features, and autoantibodies. This material is intended to be an overview, with both the concepts and specific findings to be explained in more detail in the following chapters.

Definitions: Is Sjogren's Syndrome a Disease?

Why isn't Sjogren's syndrome a disease? It really is when viewed from a current perspective. A syndrome, as defined in the *Random House Dictionary*, is "a group of symptoms that characterizes a disease," whereas a disease, according to *Stedman's Medical Dictionary*, is "a pathologic entity characterized by two of these criteria: a recognized etiologic agent, an identifiable group of signs and symptoms, or consistent anatomical alterations." Sjogren's syndrome has an identifiable group of signs and symptoms and consistent anatomical alterations.

Signs and Symptoms

What are the signs and symptoms of Sjogren's syndrome? The most distinctive ones, and those originally described by Henrik Sjogren, are dry eye and dry mouth due to a lack of tear production and a lack of saliva. The actual symptoms in the eye include a gritty sensation, the sense of a foreign body in the eye, or itching; redness; and an increased sensitivity to light that may make reading or watching television difficult. The symptoms of lack of saliva may include difficulty chewing, swallowing, and speaking, and severe, progressive dental caries. Patients

---

**TABLE 2.1   DISEASES ASSOCIATED
WITH SECONDARY SJOGREN'S**

Rheumatoid arthritis
Systemic lupus erythematosus
Scleroderma
Vasculitis
Polymyositis/dermatomyositis
Primary biliary cirrhosis

---

find they are continually sipping water. These distinctive symptoms have also been called the sicca syndrome (from the Latin *siccus,* meaning "dry").

Other organs in the body that secrete moist material, usually as a form of mucus, can also participate in this sicca syndrome and produce troublesome symptoms in patients with Sjogren's. Among these organs are the lungs, the upper airways such as the nose and throat, the vagina, and the skin. These symptoms, however, are not used to define the disease.

Finally, since Sjogren's is, as we shall see, a chronic inflammatory disease, patients complain of symptoms common to all inflammatory diseases, such as chronic and profound fatigue, as well as symptoms common to all chronic diseases, such as depression. These symptoms, while real and often disabling, are too nonspecific to define the disease.

Primary and Secondary Sjogren's

Henrik Sjogren also reported that 13 of the original 19 patients he described had arthritis. Arthritis in patients with Sjogren's resembles rheumatoid arthritis, but there is usually less swelling. On the other hand, 15–30 percent of patients with unequivocal rheumatoid arthritis may develop Sjogren's syndrome. This situation can be the source of much confusion and has led to the concept of primary and secondary Sjogren's. Patients have secondary Sjogren's when they also have another autoimmune disease—most commonly rheumatoid arthritis (RA) or systemic lupus erythematosus (SLE), but a large number of other autoimmune diseases qualify as well (Table 2.1).

Inflammation of the Glands

Patients with Sjogren's may have enlarged or swollen lacrimal or salivary glands. When one biopsies such glands and examines the tissue microscopically, one sees that the glands are infiltrated by white blood cells. These cells include B cells or antibody-producing lymphocytes, activated T lymphocytes, and macrophages. Together these cells produce a localized inflammation that is ultimately capable of destroying the gland. This inflammatory process is similar, if not identical, to that involving the islets of the pancreas in type 1 diabetes mellitus, the synovial membrane lining the joints in rheumatoid arthritis, and the tissues specifically involved in the other autoimmune diseases. The inflammatory infiltration of white blood cells can also be seen in the very small salivary glands that line the lower lip. These minor salivary glands are very easy to biopsy and are very helpful in making the diagnosis of Sjogren's. It is useful to make the diagnosis early because glands that have been invaded but not yet destroyed have enough residual glandular tissue to respond to medication that stimulates salivary flow.

Autoimmunity

Autoimmune diseases are so named because in these diseases the B lymphocytes produce antibodies to, and the T lymphocytes are activated by, proteins or protein-nucleic acid complexes that are a normal component of the body's own cells. The underlying reason for this abnormal immune response is not completely known, nor in the case of Sjogren's has the specific protein in the glandular tissue been identified for certain, but enough is known to definitely classify Sjogren's as an autoimmune disease. A hallmark of autoimmune diseases is the production of antibodies circulating in the blood that are characteristic for the specific autoimmune disease in question. This is true in Sjogren's, in which antibodies to one or both of two protein-RNA complexes, called Ro/SSA and La/SSB, are present in more than 60 percent and 40 percent, respectively, of the serum from patients with Sjogren's. These autoantibodies are also commonly found in the serum of patients with SLE, thereby strengthening the concept of Sjogren's as an autoimmune disease.

The International Classification Criteria for Sjogren's

As one can see, Sjogren's fulfills the definition of a disease. It has a definite and almost unique set of sicca symptoms, a definite anatomic-

---

TABLE 2.2   REVISED EUROPEAN-AMERICAN CRITERIA FOR THE CLASSIFICATION OF SJOGREN'S SYNDROME

---

1. Ocular symptoms (1 of 3)
   - Dry eyes for longer than three months
   - Sensation of a foreign body in the eye
   - Use of artificial tears more often than three times a day
2. Oral symptoms (1 of 3)
   - Dry mouth for longer than three months
   - Swollen salivary glands
   - Need liquids to swallow
3. Ocular tests (1 of 2)
   - Unanesthetized Schirmer's $\leqslant$ 5 mm/5 minutes
   - Vital dye staining
4. Positive lip biopsy (focus score $\geqslant$ 1/4 mm^2)
5. Oral tests (1 of 3)
   - Unstimulated salivary flow rate $\leqslant$ 0.1 ml/minute
   - Abnormal parotid sialography
   - Abnormal salivary scintigraphy
6. Positive anti-SSA and/or SSB

Diagnosis of primary Sjogren's syndrome requires 4 of 6 criteria, including item 4 or item 6. Diagnosis of secondary Sjogren's syndrome requires established connective tissue disease and one sicca symptom plus 2 of 3 objective tests for dry mouth and dry eye (items 3–5). Diagnosis of Sjogren's syndrome can be made in patients who have no sicca symptoms if 3 of the 4 objective tests are fulfilled (items 3–6).
Modified from *Ann Rheum Dis*, 2002; 61:554–558.

pathologic basis, and a well-defined pair of autoantibodies. Still, Sjogren's is not easy to diagnose and until very recently was not easy to define in a way that would enable patients with Sjogren's to be studied as a uniform group. Thus an international committee of experts was assembled, under the auspices of the Sjogren's Syndrome Foundation, to formulate diagnostic criteria so that patients who could be universally considered to have Sjogren's could be entered into clinical trials and other forms of research (Table 2.2). These classification criteria, published in 2002, now define how one decides that a patient has unequivocal Sjogren's. Early in the disease, patients who actually have Sjogren's may not meet all of the criteria, so bear in mind that the diagnosis and treatment of any individual patient is a matter of clinical judgment.

It is important to rule out diseases that might also produce typical Sjogren's findings. These conditions include:

- Previous radiation to the head and neck

- Lymphoma

- Sarcoidosis

- Hepatitis C infection

- HIV infection (AIDS)

- Graft-versus-host disease

- Medications that can cause dryness

Summing Up

Sjogren's is a relatively common and serious autoimmune disease that involves an inflammatory immune destruction of the lacrimal and salivary glands, producing a well-defined set of symptoms connected with dry mouth and dry eye. Constitutional symptoms such as fatigue, joint pain, and depression are also common.

3 Who Develops Sjogren's Syndrome?

SINCE SJOGREN'S IS A SYNDROME and a disease, ascertaining how many people have it and elucidating its epidemiologic features have proven to be difficult undertakings. Although there are a variety of reasons for this, the most important is that an international consensus on how to define Sjogren's has only recently been agreed upon. This chapter will review how many people have Sjogren's and the principal identifying features of those individuals, as well as issues relating to genetic predisposition.

How Many People Have Sjogren's?

Most professionals trained in estimating the numbers of people with a disorder do so in terms of prevalence or incidence. Prevalence is defined as the number of individuals per 100,000 people with a condition, while incidence is the number per 100,000 who are diagnosed in a given year. Some papers have published figures based upon self-reported dry eye or dry mouth with arthritis. Others have relied upon older definitions of Sjogren's, which could include dry eye, dry mouth, and arthritis as a consequence of viral infections such as AIDS or hepatitis. If we restrict ourselves to autoimmune Sjogren's, the Sjogren's Syndrome Foundation estimates that 4 million people in the United States (out of 280 million) have it. This breaks down to one person in 70.

Where did these numbers come from? In the United States, approximately 0.5 percent of the population, or 1 person in 200, meets the criteria for primary Sjogren's. To these 1.4 million Americans, we next add the numbers who fulfill the criteria for other autoimmune conditions and who also have Sjogren's. Since approximately 30 percent overall with rheumatoid arthritis (3 million), systemic lupus erythematosus (1 million), and scleroderma-related disorders and other musculoskeletal conditions that are autoimmune diseases (1 million) also fulfill definitions for Sjogren's, 1.5 million of these 5 million bring the total to 2.9 million. How does one account for the remaining 1.1 million? Simply because Sjogren's is underreported. Many people (especially with mild Sjogren's) never bother to complain to their doctor about their symptoms, or their health care professional lacks the education and experience to make a diagnosis.

Age, Race, Geography, Sex, and the Environment
The mean age of onset of Sjogren's is in the early 50s. Less than 5 percent of Sjogren's patients are under the age of 20, and nearly all of these have anti-Ro/SSA antibodies. Sjogren's syndrome is probably found in all races and ethnicities to a similar extent, although this has not been well studied. In the last decade, published studies estimating the prevalence of the syndrome in China, Spain, Slovenia, Finland, Greece, and the United States have demonstrated strikingly similar results. In all these surveys, 90–95 percent of people with primary Sjogren's were female. The percentage is slightly lower in secondary disease, but for all practical purposes signs and symptoms of Sjogren's in males and females are the same. Hormonal influences no doubt play a role in female predominance of the syndrome, but this issue has not been adequately explored.

While chemical or environmental exposures play a role in other rheumatic disorders associated with Sjogren's syndrome, except for sun sensitivity (which is directly related to antibodies to anti-Ro/SSA), no specific chemical or occupational endeavor correlates with its presence. One exception would be increased symptoms of Sjogren's syndrome among individuals residing in regions with a dry climate.

Primary and Secondary Sjogren's
Patients with primary Sjogren's by definition lack the obvious distinguishing features of rheumatoid arthritis, systemic lupus erythematosus, or scleroderma (see Chapter 11). These include deforming arthritis, discoid rashes, and tight skin. However, compared to individuals with secondary Sjogren's, there are certain features noted more commonly in primary Sjogren's. These consist of Raynaud's phenomenon (color

changes in the hands with cold exposure), salivary gland enlargement, swollen lymph nodes, anti-Ro/SSA and anti-La/SSB positivity, central nervous system dysfunction, and the potential for developing lymphoma (44 times greater than in healthy individuals).

Sjogren's, Genetics, and Other Autoimmune Diseases

Sjogren's syndrome can run in families. One Sjogren's patient in eight will have a relative (usually female) with the condition. Only a handful of reports of identical twins with Sjogren's have been published; clearly the genetics of the syndrome are complex and multifactorial. A first-degree relative (parent, sibling, or child) of someone with Sjogren's has a 1–3 percent risk of developing the syndrome. Actually, these relatives have a much higher risk for being diagnosed with autoimmune thyroid disease or lupus than Sjogren's. In some studies, up to 30 percent of Sjogren's patients have Hashimoto's thryoiditis or are hypothyroid. Other autoimmune conditions found in 1–30 percent of Sjogren's patients include lupus, rheumatoid arthritis, scleroderma, inflammatory myositis, type 1 diabetes, and multiple sclerosis. Occasionally, family members of Sjogren's patients have antinuclear antibodies, rheumatoid factor, and anti-Ro/SSA on blood testing without any symptoms of or evidence for autoimmune disease. A variety of genetic markers on the surface of cells known as human leukocyte antigen (HLA) haplotypes also predispose individuals to Sjogren's. These are reviewed in Chapters 4 and 5.

Summing Up

One American in 70 has Sjogren's, evenly divided between primary and secondary disease. This population is overwhelmingly female and middle-aged. Sjogren's patients present an increased risk of having another autoimmune disorder, a family member with autoimmune disease, and lymphoma. No geographic, racial, environmental, or ethnic risk factors have been associated with primary Sjogren's syndrome.

PART II

The Pathology of Sjogren's Syndrome

What goes awry in our body that creates the symptoms and signs of Sjogren's syndrome? In this section, we learn that Sjogren's results from a dysfunctional immune system, which leads to inflammation and the formation of autoantibodies. This is compounded by a pathologic process resulting in dryness.

This section of the handbook is not an easy read. Indeed, many rheumatologists and immunologists have difficulty grappling with these concepts. However, we have tried to present complex concepts in a relatively easy-to-understand fashion.

Janine Smith, MD

Serena Morrison, MD

4 What Leads to Dryness?

SJOGREN'S SYNDROME affects the exocrine glands, which produce saliva and tears. Two of the key features of Sjogren's syndrome are dry eye (also called keratoconjunctivitis sicca or KCS) and dry mouth (also called xerostomia). What is the cause of this dryness? In this chapter, the normal function and disease-related dysfunction of the lacrimal and salivary glands affected in Sjogren's syndrome will be discussed. Then theories about the cause of the dryness will be considered.

The Lacrimal Gland

Since the source of human tears is the lacrimal gland, it is important to know its normal anatomy and structure. The lacrimal gland is located underneath the upper eyelid on the outer side near the temple. There are two lobes of the lacrimal gland, the palpebral and the orbital. Some smaller, accessory lacrimal glands are located on the conjunctiva (the transparent membrane that covers the white part of the eye and which gets red when irritated) (Table 4.1).

The lacrimal glands should constantly be producing tears while we are performing our normal activities. Their purpose is to lubricate and protect the surface of the eye. We are usually unaware of these tears, called basal tears. Reflex or emergency tears are produced to flush and lubricate the eye quickly if a particle or chemical gets into the eye, or by emotion. Some people with dry eye have painful episodes due to decreased amounts of basal tears, but because their lacrimal gland is not completely damaged, they can still produce a normal amount of reflex tears. They may even think they have excess tearing when in fact they have dry eye. This is because as their eyes dry out from a lack of basal

---

TABLE 4.1   EXOCRINE GLANDS

---

1. Lacrimal glands (produces tears)
   a. Consists of palpebral lobe, orbital lobe, and accessory glands
   b. Tear film layers: mucous, aqueous, lipid
2. Salivary glands (produces saliva)
   a. Consists of parotid, submandibular, and sublingual glands
   b. Secretions (mucous and serous)

---

tears, their eyes start to hurt, and this triggers a large amount of emergency tears. One of the signs of severe damage to the lacrimal gland is an inability to cry emotional or emergency tears.

In Sjogren's syndrome, the lacrimal gland does not produce a sufficient volume of tear fluid. In addition, the tears produced are abnormal in their consistency and do not lubricate or protect the surface of the eye well. For example, the tears are unstable and often evaporate faster than normal, leaving dry spots on the surface of the eye (see "Tear Film Layers," below); people often feel as though their eyes are driest at the end of the day. In addition, when reading or concentrating (such as when working on a computer), people blink less, which allows the tear film to evaporate more readily. Dry eye can result in a decreased ability to read for extended periods of time.

Tear Film Maintenance

Before delving into the components of the tears, it is important to mention the role of the eyelids and cornea in maintaining the tear layer. Blinking spreads the tears over the eye and pushes debris toward the inner corner of the eye so that it can drain into the nose through a small opening in the eyelid, called the punctum. This is why mucus collects in the corner of the eye.

Any malfunction in eyelid movement or decreased frequency of blinking (as occurs with tasks that require visual attention, such as reading or using the computer) can worsen dry eye symptoms. The cornea is like the crystal on a watch. It is the transparent covering of the center portion of the outer surface of the eye. Along with the tears, the cornea functions as a lens to make vision sharp and clear. If the cornea is not smooth—say, because of dryness—the tears are not well distributed, and blurred vision can result.

Tear Film Layers

Tears have three major components: mucous, aqueous (or liquid), and lipid (or oily). These contents are arranged in layers, and the components of each layer must be healthy and in balance for the tears to function properly.

The *mucous layer* is the tear layer that is closest to the eye surface. Special cells that are found in the conjunctiva, called goblet cells, create mucin, which makes up this layer. This layer makes the tears slippery and anchors them loosely to the surface of the cornea for protection. It also helps prevent infection by keeping bacteria from sticking to the surface of the eye.

The *aqueous layer* is the liquid component of the tears and hydrates the mucous layer to form a sort of tear gel. This layer is produced by the lacrimal gland and also lubricates and enhances the spreadability of the tear film. The aqueous layer contains proteins such as lysozyme and lactoferrin, which act like antibiotics and protect the eye from bacteria.

Tiny sebaceous (oil-producing) glands, called Meibomian glands, are located along the margin of the eyelids, adjacent to the lashes. They produce the *lipid layer* of the tear film, which enhances tear stability and retards evaporation of the tears. If the lipid layer is completely removed, the rate of evaporation is increased fourfold.

Salivary Glands

Sjogren's syndrome also affects the salivary glands. The principal glands of salivation are the parotid, submandibular, and sublingual glands, which are located in the cheek, under the chin, and under the tongue, respectively. When these glands are functioning well, they can produce 800–1,500 milliliters of saliva each day.

These glands produce two major types of secretions. The first is the serous secretion, which contains ptyalin. Ptyalin is an enzyme that helps digest starches. The second type is the mucous secretion, which contains mucin for lubricating and protection.

So what is so important about saliva? The mouth is loaded with bacteria that can cause infection, destroy tissue, and promote cavities (dental caries). The saliva helps wash away the bacteria and food particles that the bacteria require to survive. Several factors within the saliva even destroy bacteria.

Both the eye and the mouth encounter bacteria and environmental irritants on an ongoing basis. Both the eyes and mouth need lubrication, since they are constantly in motion. Saliva and tears contain all the necessary elements to protect and lubricate the surfaces of the eyes and mouth.

Theories of How Sjogren's Syndrome Develops

The production of tears and saliva is complicated. There are many steps involved in the production of these complex fluids, and disruption of this process can reduce the amount of the secretions and alter their composition. Nerve fibers going into the glands, the acinar gland cells (which are the cells that produce the fluid), the stromal cells (which support the acinar cells), and even sex hormones all play a major role in the production of saliva and tears. All aspects of these systems need to be functioning and in concert with each other for normal tear and saliva production.

Decrease in Glandular Cell Output

The lacrimal and salivary glands are exocrine glands. This means that they have special cells, acinar cells, that empty into the body through ducts that produce secretions. In order for the acinar cells to make liquid, their relationship with the supporting stromal cells needs to be just right. If this relationship is disrupted, secretion will decline.

Damage to these special gland cells can occur with an autoimmune event. In these cases, for some unknown reason, the body's lymphocytes (the body's immune defense cells) are attracted to the salivary and lacrimal glands. Once the lymphocytes gather in the exocrine glands, they multiply and become the focus of inflammation. This inflammation is an attack by the body on itself. For example, the lymphocytes release compounds called cytokines that can injure the acinar cells and can even cause the stromal cells to dysfunction and fail to support the acinar cells. As a result, the gland cells become sick and can even die. When an acinar cell dies, it releases its contents, which are recognized as foreign, and the process can lead to even more inflammation. Sick gland cells do not produce normal amounts or quality of fluid secretions.

Nerve Destruction

Normally messages sent through the nerve fibers to an exocrine gland cause it to produce fluid. Damage to or dysfunction of the nerves can lead to surface dryness by disturbing the fluid production and release. The salivary and lacrimal glands have a direct link to the brain through these nerve fibers. Think of the brain as central command and the nerves that link the brain and the glands as the messengers.

In one scenario, the central command (brain) gets confused; even though it senses that tears or saliva need to be produced, it sends out the wrong signal, and the tears and saliva are not made. Drugs can also cause this confusion at the brain level. That is why many medicines often have the side effect of dry mouth and dry eye.

The second situation is that the central command knows exactly what needs to happen and sends the correct message through the messengers (nerves), but it is the messengers that are confused this time. One possibility is that products of inflammation called cytokines cause paralysis in these nerves. The result is that the glands that are supposed to be stimulated fail to receive the message to make tears and saliva, although they are capable of doing so.

A third possibility involves the cornea (the surface of the eye) and its connection to the neural centers. If for some reason the cornea's nerves are not working well, then no message will be sent to the brain that tears are needed. Without the message that a problem exists, the brain does not know to send a message to the lacrimal gland to increase secretions. Any interruption of this feedback loop, which some researchers call a servomechanism, can decrease the amount of secretions.

Sex Hormones

Another factor to be considered is the role of sex hormones. It is known that autoimmunity is more prevalent in women than men. Could this be because of the sex hormones? Women normally have higher levels of estrogen and lower levels of androgens than men, and eye tissue has components that specifically bind to sex hormones. It has been found that with a decrease in local androgens, the inflammation mentioned above goes unchecked. A certain amount of androgens are required to maintain a noninflamed state in exocrine glands. For example, androgens decrease the production of autoantibodies, and estrogens tend to promote inflammation. Some studies have even found that hormone replacement therapy (with estrogen and progestin) is associated with dry eye in postmenopausal women.

Autoimmune Theories

In the foregoing section, we talked about how damage to the lacrimal and salivary glands, a problem with the nervous system, or a disturbance in the level or balance of sex hormones could result in dryness. One prevalent theme for the cause of the damage is autoimmunity. But what triggers the autoimmunity? Scientists are investigating many theories: that the cause of Sjogren's syndrome may be an infectious trigger, a genetic factor, a combination of factors, or a cause that we have not even considered.

Extension of the Inflammatory Theory: Apoptosis

Apoptosis is the process by which a cell is programmed to self-destruct. If the cells do not die when they are supposed to, problems result. Cells that keep growing and dividing can become tumors and may be malignant. What does this have to do with Sjogren's syndrome? In Sjogren's, when the lymphocytes arrive at the fluid-producing lacrimal or salivary gland, instead of just passing through, they are activated and signal the immune system to initiate an attack. That is a problem in itself. The second problem is that the lymphocytes are supposed to die at some point but sometimes do not undergo natural death or apoptosis. The lymphocytes accumulate in the glands and keep stimulating the immune system to attack the glands. An accumulation of lymphocytes, called a focus of inflammation, is characteristic in exocrine glands of people with Sjogren's syndrome. This focus is what is found when a lip biopsy of a minor salivary gland is performed in the diagnosis of Sjogren's syndrome. An increased risk for Sjogren's syndrome may exist in people whose cells are resistant to apoptosis.

Infections: Viral, Epstein-Barr-like, or H. pylori

Infection with viruses such as hepatitis C, human lymphotrophic leukemia virus (HTLV-1), and human immunodeficiency virus (HIV) has been known to cause dry eye. Therefore, viral infection in general (not necessarily with the above viruses) has been identified as a potential pathogenic mechanism for Sjogren's syndrome.

When viruses enter a person's body they can change the surfaces of the normal cells so that the cells look like foreign invaders such as bacteria. As a result of changes in these markers, the cells are no longer recognized as self, and the body's defenses attack them as if they were a foreign invader.

Another mechanism involves invading microbes, which sneak past the body's defenses by disguising themselves as native cells. If the defenses figure out this plan, they attack the invaders. Unfortunately, the native cells are so similar to the microbes that the defense cells cannot differentiate and therefore attack the native cells as well.

Epstein-Barr virus (EBV) is implicated as a contributor to Sjogren's syndrome. The picture is not clear, and the only evidence is indirect. EBV is a very common virus in the herpes family, and almost everyone has had it at some point. Usually EBV infection is very mild. Most people get flulike symptoms and swollen parotid glands but quickly recover. A few people get more serious symptoms from EBV such as fatigue and swollen lymph glands (including the spleen). This type of infection with EBV is a condition called infectious mononucleosis. The virus enters the salivary glands, which swell and can become painful.

The interesting part about EBV is that after its initial infection, it quiets down and hides away. It tends to be dormant in the salivary gland. Once in a while the EBV can be reactivated. This often happens only when the person has immune system suppression (e.g., a patient who chemotherapy and does not have normal defenses). If the virus reactivates, it can trigger chronic inflammation (by revving up the immune system), and an example of uncontrolled inflammation could be Sjogren's syndrome. No conclusive evidence proves this theory correct, but it is a possibility. Questions remain: since most people have EBV, why do some reactivate, and why does this reactivation trigger inflammation? Genetic background may be an important factor in determining who is susceptible to a viral infection triggering an abnormal inflammatory response.

Some researchers are looking for an association between *Helicobacter pylori* and Sjogren's syndrome. *H. pylori* is more commonly known as the bacterium that causes stomach ulcers. Interestingly, *H. pylori* is being recognized as the cause of infections in many other parts of the body as well.

A lot of controversy exists as to whether *H. pylori* plays any role in the development of Sjogren's syndrome. Some studies found an increased prevalence of *H. pylori* infections in Sjogren's syndrome patients, but other studies could not confirm this. The trouble with this research is that once *H. pylori* triggers an infection, it is often difficult to detect at a later time. Further research into the role of *H. pylori* infection in Sjogren's syndrome is ongoing.

Genetics

As mentioned above, the environment (such as viruses and bacteria) is a consideration for the cause of Sjogren's syndrome, but another big factor is the person's genetic background. Does something about the genetic makeup of someone with Sjogren's syndrome make that person more susceptible to autoimmune disease? For unknown reasons, some patterns of genes make certain people more susceptible than others to autoimmune diseases such as Sjogren's syndrome. When a certain mix occurs between the genes and the environment, then autoimmune diseases can be triggered.

For example, each gland cell has a protein on its surface: a human leukocyte antigen (HLA). Think of this as the gland cell's identification card. People have a certain type of HLA on all of their cells, including those in the exocrine glands. These HLA types have been labeled as HLA-DR1, HLA-DR2, and so on. All the different HLA types should signal that the gland cell is friendly to the lymphocyte. But for some unknown reason, the lymphocytes sometimes get confused when reading the HLA-DR3 gene in Caucasians, which results in a higher incidence of Sjogren's syndrome in this race. The HLA-DR3 antigen is most often found in patients who develop antibodies to Ro/SSA or La/SSB. Interestingly, HLA-DR3 in other races does not seem to have the same effect; other HLA-DR genes trigger Sjogren's syndrome in other races.

ICA-69

As another example, ICA-69 is a recently identified self-antigen, or component of a specific tissue or cell that is being mistakenly recognized as foreign by the immune system. The actual function of ICA-69 is unknown, but it is known to act as a self-antigen in the salivary glands, lacrimal glands, pancreatic cells, and nervous system tissue. It may have been altered by infection or inflammation or it may be in its natural form. An example of this was mentioned above in the virus section. As a virus invades the body, it can cause changes in native cells and create a self-antigen. The native cells are then no longer recognized by the body's defense system, a fact that leads to self-attack.

Of interest is that some patients with Sjogren's syndrome develop complications involving the nervous system. Autoimmune targeting of ICA-69 may play a role in this process, since ICA-69 is also expressed in nervous tissue.

Summing Up

In this chapter the normal function of the exocrine glands affected by Sjogren's syndrome has been detailed. An intricate pathway exists to create the right amount, components and consistency of tears and saliva. If this process is disrupted in any way, the production and components of the secretions can be altered. We know an autoimmune process is involved, but many possibilities exist as to why Sjogren's syndrome starts and how it damages the body. The cause of the body's attack on itself remains unclear, and a combination of infection and genetics is being investigated as a potential disease-inducing factor.

With further research, the answer may be revealed to be one of the proposed theories, but more likely it will be some combination of these factors. Inflammation clearly results in malfunction of the fluid-producing glands, but the cause of the inflammation is unclear. For now, the exact cause of the Sjogren's syndrome remains unknown.

Lama Hashish, MD

Amr Sawalha, MD

John B. Harley, MD, PhD

Robert Fox, MD, PhD

5 Sjogren's Syndrome: A Genetic and Immunologic Perspective

SJOGREN'S SYNDROME is an autoimmune disorder that presents when one's genetic predisposition combines with environmental or infectious factors. Further, there are neural and hormonal influences. This chapter reviews how these factors interact with the immune system to produce Sjogren's syndrome.

The Genetics of Sjogren's

Several genetic and environmental factors are involved in the pathogenesis of primary Sjogren's syndrome. Indeed, interaction between susceptibility genes and the various environmental factors are thought to define the conditions that make this disease possible. Similar to many other autoimmune disorders, Sjogren's syndrome appears to be a complicated disease with many different susceptibility genes and environmental factors, most of which are unknown.

The evidence for genetic susceptibility was first recognized in a family that had Sjogren's syndrome involving three generations at once; the case was published in 1937. More recent advances in genetics research methodology have allowed the identification of strong associations with human histocompatibility antigen (HLA) as well as other genes. (The HLA allele associations that have been replicated, and thus confirmed, include HLA-DRB1*0301, HLA-DRB1*1501, HLA-DQA1*0103, HLA-DQA1*0501, HLA-DQB1*0201, and HLA-DQB1*0601.)

24

**TABLE 5.1   IMPORTANT COMPONENTS OF THE IMMUNE
                  SYSTEM IN SJOGREN'S SYNDROME**

---

1. White blood cells
   a. Granulocytes—promote acute inflammation
   b. Lymphocytes—promote chronic inflammation
      i.   T cells (memory cells)
      ii. B cells (promote production of autoantibodies)
2. Proteins
   a. Albumin—carrier proteins, decreased in chronic disease
   b. Globulin—levels increased in inflammation
      i.   Alpha globulins
      ii.   Beta globulins
      iii. Gamma globulins—IgG, IgM, IgD, IgA, and IgE
3. Important autoantibodies in Sjogren's
   a. Anti-Ro/SSA
   b. Anti-La/SSB
   c. Rheumatoid factor
   d. Antinuclear antibody
   e. Anti-muscarinic receptor antibody

Mutations in various cytokines (which act as cell messengers) and related genes have also been associated with primary Sjogren's syndrome. Examples include interleukin-10 (IL-10) and interleukin-6 (IL-6). Other genetic associations reported include polymorphisms in the complement component mannose-binding lectin (MBL), tumor necrosis factor-alpha (TNF-α), and transporters associated with antigen processing (TAP2). In addition, mutations in Ro52 and glutathione S-transferase M1 (GSTM1) genes have been reported. The individual role of each of these genes in Sjogren's syndrome is yet to be understood.

The Pathogenic Role of Autoantibodies in Sjogren's

It is thought that the pathogenesis of this disorder includes two processes. There is a T-lymphocyte-mediated process that leads to direct cell destruction and a B-lymphocyte activation process that leads to the production of the autoantibodies (see Table 5.1 and Figure 5.1).

Destruction of the salivary and lacrimal glands and other target tissues is attributed to focal lymphocytic infiltration, which involves primarily T-lymphocytes (a kind of white blood cell that plays a role in immune system function).

There are a number of different kinds of autoantibodies in Sjogren's syndrome. Antibodies are proteins that we make to defend against all

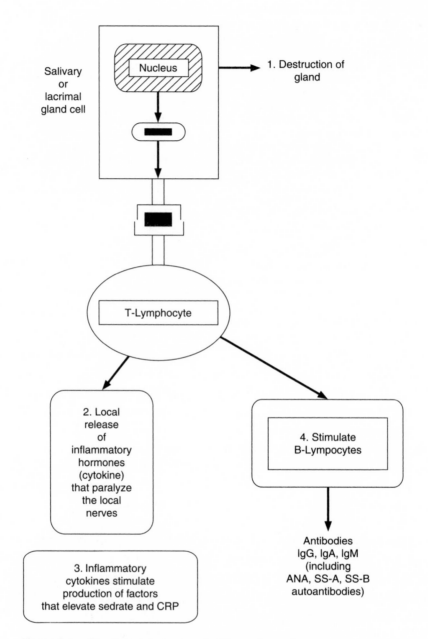

Figure 5.1. The immune response in Sjogren's syndrome

kinds of different infections. They are also called immunoglobulins and have a few major types: IgG, IgM, IgA, and IgE. (Immunoglobulin E causes many kinds of allergy.) Antibodies are not usually supposed to bind to something that we are made of. When they do, they are called *autoantibodies*. Most of the known autoantibodies in Sjogren's are of the IgG type, though at least some are IgA.

Autoantibodies have names that tell us what they bind to, but this does not reveal what they do or how they work. Anti-Ro/SSA, anti-La/SSB, rheumatoid factor, antinuclear antibody, and anti-muscarinic receptor are found in the bloodstream of a substantial fraction of Sjogren's syndrome patients. The finding of an autoantibody is frequently an indication that the immune system may be involved in the disease process. There is some evidence that these autoantibodies are important pathogenic factors in damage to target organs as well as the extraglandular manifestations.

The antibodies most commonly looked for are the antinuclear antibody (ANA) and the Sjogren's-associated antibodies, anti-Ro/SSA and anti-La/SSB; the latter two are even used in the recent diagnostic criteria. However, there is a great deal of confusion about the meaning of a positive antibody (especially if it is weak) and if Sjogren's can exist if the antibody is negative. There is a common misunderstanding that antinuclear antibodies are both sensitive and specific. In fact, there is a relatively high frequency of antinuclear autoantibodies in otherwise healthy individuals, patients with liver disease, and patients with carcinoma. The frequency of ANA in putatively normal individuals can be as high as 31.7 percent of individuals at a 1:40 serum dilution, 13.3 percent at 1:80, 5.0 percent at 1:160, and 3.3 percent at 1:320. However, it has been calculated that the risk of an individual with ANA 1:320 developing systemic lupus erythematosus or Sjogren's during a ten-year follow-up period is less than 5 percent.

The role of antibodies against nuclear antigens (ANA) as well as anti-Ro/SSA and anti-La/SSB in the pathogenesis of Sjogren's has always been puzzling, since these antigens are found in all nucleated cells. The purpose of the immune system has always been assumed to distinguish self from non-self in a strict manner. Until relatively recently, it was assumed that the body did not generate antibodies against its own antigens. However, we now recognize that the body continually makes an initial response against many self-antigens, but at a low level. This is reflected in the high frequency of low-titer autoantibodies described above and the observation that most patients with a higher-titer ANA (such as ANA 1:320) do not actually go on to get Sjogren's or lupus. The key question then becomes why some of these anti-self responses escalate and contribute to disease, while other anti-self immune reactions just go away.

Anti-muscarinic receptor antibody is the most interesting from the perspective of current thinking. This antibody is thought to block the action of the nerves that go to the salivary and lacrimal glands, thereby reducing the production of saliva and tears. The detection of anti-muscarinic receptor antibodies is very difficult and is performed in only a few research laboratories around the world.

The primary cause of Sjogren's syndrome has not been identified, but as noted above, several factors are thought to contribute to the pathogenesis of this disorder. Those factors are genetic and environmental, including hormone effects and viral infections.

Hormonal Influences

Estrogen activity may be involved in developing dry mouth and dry eye symptoms because of the following factors:

- Sjogren's affects women much more frequently than men.

- The symptoms of dry mouth and dry eye are more prevalent in patients who are receiving hormone replacement therapy than those who are not.

Viruses, the Immune System, and Sjogren's

It is thought that some viral infections could have a role in the pathogenesis of Sjogren's syndrome by the following mechanism. After a virus or bacterium enters the body, an immune reaction is almost always activated. (Parasitic infections are less of a threat to us than they were to our forebears.) Thankfully, the infection is almost always defeated and the person returns to normal health. Sometimes this initial response against the virus or bacterium becomes chronic because the body cannot clear the infection, and sometimes the immune response heads off in the direction of autoimmunity. Examples of infections that can cause chronic problems include streptococci (a bacterium that can cause rheumatic fever), human immunodeficiency virus (HIV), and hepatitis C virus (chronic hepatitis). Indeed, hepatitis C virus can cause dry eye, dry mouth, and arthritis, all symptoms found in Sjogren's syndrome.

Epstein-Barr Virus

Epstein-Barr virus has been suggested as a possible activator or co-factor in the development of Sjogren's syndrome. Once we are infected with this virus, we remain infected for the rest of our lives, and nearly everyone is infected. The evidence for this virus being important in Sjogren's syndrome has not yet convinced most scientists, and it remains an idea that is not generally accepted.

Hepatitis C

Chronic hepatitis C can cause symptoms that are similar to Sjogren's syndrome (dry mouth, dry eye, and arthritis, occurring in association with an enlarged parotid gland with lymphocytic infiltration). Anti-Ro/SSA and anti-La/SSB, which are present in the sera of Sjogren's syndrome patients, are typically absent in the sera of the patient with chronic hepatitis C infection, as are the usual pathologic findings of autoimmune Sjogren's syndrome. Most experts in Sjogren's syndrome lean toward including hepatitis C as one of the differential diagnoses of dry eye-dry mouth syndrome, as other features distinguish it.

Retroviruses

Two retroviruses, human immunodeficiency virus (HIV) and human T-cell leukemia virus (HTLV-1), are known to be causes of a syndrome that presents with a clinical picture similar to that seen in Sjogren's syndrome. Those viruses affect males more than females, and the autoantibodies that define Sjogren's syndrome have not been found in the patients who carry those viruses. HLTV-1 may cause muscle deterioration and causes a condition with the unattractive name of tropical spastic paraparesis. This virus is endemic in some parts of the world.

The medical literature now has many, many reports describing the dry eye and mouth associated with HIV infection. Both Sjogren's and HIV infection have diffuse lymphocyte infiltration in the affected tissues. However, the kind of lymphocyte that dominates in HIV-infected patients tends to be different than those that dominate in Sjogren's syndrome. The characteristic autoantibodies, anti-Ro/SSA and anti-La/SSB, are typically not found in HIV-infected patients. There are other gene-related differences as well. Consequently, HIV-infected patients are not usually considered to have Sjogren's syndrome, but there is some disagreement among doctors on this point.

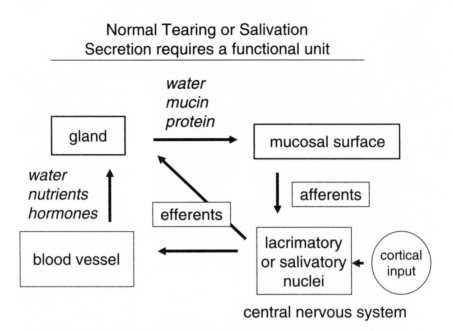

Figure 5.2. Normal Tearing or Salivation Secretion requires a functional unit

Background: The Functional Circuit That Links Ocular/ Oral Symptoms and Secretory Function

In order to understand the spectrum of disorders that contribute to dry eye and mouth, it is important to recognize that these symptoms result from an imbalance in a functional circuit that controls lacrimal and salivary function. The functional circuit can be considered to start at the mucosal membrane (either the ocular surface or buccal mucosal surface) where the patient has decreased aqueous secretions (Figure 5.2). These highly innervated surfaces send unmyelinated nerves to specific regions of the midbrain, termed the lacrimatory and salvatory nuclei. This midbrain region sends signals to the cortex, where dryness is sensed, and receives input from cortical centers that reflect input such as depression or stress reactions associated with dryness. The clearest evidence of these cortical inputs is the classical Pavlovian response of salivation in response to other cortical stimuli. After the midbrain receives input from the mucosa and higher cortical centers, efferent (outgoing) nerves that innervate the glands using cholinergic neurotransmitters (especially acetylcholine and vasoactive intestinal peptide) and blood vessels using adrenergic (adrenalin-containing) neurotransmitters are activated. The presence of inflammatory infiltrates in the glands contributes to inade-

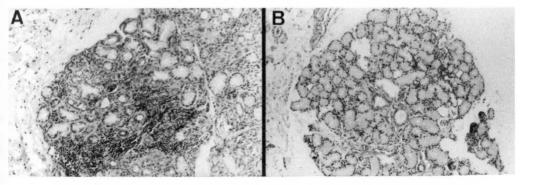

Figure 5.3. A salivary gland seen in a patient with Sjogren's syndrome demonstrating inflammation (A), as compared with a normal gland (B).

quate secretory response not only by destruction of glandular elements but also by interfering with effective release of neurotransmitters by the nerves in the end organ and the response of the glandular cells at the level of post-receptor signaling. As a result, there is decreased activation of the receptors that subsequently produce the energy source for water transport. Thus, a key point in the pathogenesis of Sjogren's is the observation that the salivary and lacrimal glands are not totally destroyed and local immune-generated release of cytokines, autoantibodies, and other chemicals leads to dysfunction of the residual glands.

Although rheumatologists are talking about autoantibodies and acute phase reactants, the patient has complaints about dry, painful eyes and mouth. In the initial stages of the disorder, patients are describing increased friction as the upper eyelid traverses the globe or the tongue moves over the buccal mucosa. For example, the upper eyelid normally traverses the globe on a carpet of lubricating tear film, composed of a mixture of aqueous and mucous secretions. When the aqueous tear or saliva component is deficient, the patient senses increased friction. The friction between the upper lids can be great enough so the surface components of the conjunctiva adhere to the upper lid and are torn off by upper-lid motion. Defects of the surface mucin layer are detected by the retention of rose bengal, which is a characteristic test for keratoconjunctivitis sicca (dry eye). The ocular surface becomes a site of chronic inflammation, similar to a wound. From these regions arise unmyelin-ated afferent (incoming) nerves, which eventually end in specific regions of the midbrain, including the lacrimatory/salvatory nuclei. Neural signals are subsequently sent to the cortex, where pain is sensed.

In summary, symptoms of dryness can result from disruption of any portion of the functional circuit. In Sjogren's syndrome, the dryness in part results from autoimmune destruction of the salivary gland (which we see as an abnormal Sjogren's lip biopsy in Figure 5.3). However, dryness can also result from increased evaporative loss from the surface of the eye (termed non-Sjogren's keratoconjunctivitis sicca), or a sensation of dryness that originates from imbalance of neurotransmitters within the centers of the brain that control tear and/or saliva function. The latter causes of dryness, termed *central,* can include drugs with anti-cholinergic side effects, including over-the-counter cold remedies (e.g., antihistamines) and sleeping aids as well as medications used for conditions of depression or neuropathy (including amitriptyline or nortriptyline), for muscle spasm, for blood pressure, or to control seizures. Also, a variety of poorly understood processes that may influence the production of neurotransmitters in the brain including demyelinating disorders such as multiple sclerosis, depression, the process of aging, and even Alzheimer's disease, and the symptom complex termed fibromyalgia may lead to dryness by affecting the centers of the brain that control salivation and tearing or the sensation of these problems by the higher brain cortical centers.

Summing Up

Sjogren's syndrome results from the interaction of genetic and environmental factors. It is likely that multiple genes interact to predispose an individual to Sjogren's syndrome. However, even when all of the genes are present (as in identical twins), it is clear that other (presumed) environmental factors play a role, since less than 20 percent of identical twins are concordant for the disorder. No single environmental agent has been identified despite an intensive 20-year search. It is more likely that many different agents can stimulate the innate immune system, which is a primitive immune system, and thus prime the more sophisticated acquired immune system to perpetuate the autoimmune process. The molecules that define the innate system and the acquired immune system and that link the two systems are the subject of intensive research. It is hoped that an understanding of these molecular events will lead to a new generation of therapies for patients.

PART III

Where and How Can the Body be Affected by Sjogren's?

Sjogren's syndrome can affect just about any part of the body. Although most patients are aware of its impact on the eyes, ears, nose, and throat, pathologic changes occur in the heart, lung, kidney, liver, skin, and joints. Sjogren's is also associated with other rheumatic conditions. Part 3 takes the reader on a tour of the body and shows how Sjogren's can affect different tissues. This is followed by an exploration of the testing that can confirm the diagnosis, and a discussion of conditions that mimic Sjogren's.

Nehad R. Soloman, MD

Steven E. Carsons, MD

6 Generalized Symptoms and Signs of Sjogren's Syndrome

IT HAS BEEN LONG realized that Sjogren's syndrome is a complex disease, with the principal symptoms being dry eye and dry mouth. Over the course of many years it has been realized that there are a myriad of extraglandular symptoms encompassed by this disorder. These may include constitutional symptoms such as fatigue, achiness, fever, adenopathy (swollen glands), myalgias (muscle pain), and weight loss. Dryness in this disease is predominantly of the eyes and mouth, but it is not limited to these areas and commonly occurs in the skin, respiratory tract, and vaginal lining. Patients with Sjogren's syndrome may also suffer from shortness of breath, cough, joint pain and swelling, rashes, reflux, muscle weakness, urinary dysfunction, peripheral or central nervous system disease, thyroid disease, and even depression. This chapter will provide a brief overview, with focus on the various extraglandular signs and symptoms associated with Sjogren's syndrome (Table 6.1), whereas the next chapters will focus on specific organ manifestations.

Constitutional symptoms are common in Sjogren's syndrome and may be in part due to the general immune response and persistent inflammation. High levels of autoantibodies circulating in the body mediate this inflammatory immune response.

Skin Problems

The skin is a common site for signs of Sjogren's syndrome. Some symptoms and signs involving the skin include dry skin as well as a

---

TABLE 6.1   GENERAL EXTRAGLANDULAR
SYMPTOMS AND SIGNS OF
SJOGREN'S SYNDROME

Symptoms	Signs
Fatigue	Adenopathy
Myalgias	Rash
Fever	Mouth sores
Cough	Raynaud's phenomenon
Shortness of breath	Weight loss
Dysphagia	Synovitis
Reflux	Diminished reflexes
Neuropathy	Purpura
Vaginal dryness	Cracked skin
Dysuria	Hives
Achiness	Vasculitis
Joint pain	Pneumonitis
Muscle weakness	Hypokalemia
Numbness	
Tingling	
Depression	
Itchy skin	
Epigastric pain	
Nocturia	
Renal colic	
Painful intercourse	

---

whole host of rashes and discoloration. When the glands in the skin are affected by Sjogren's syndrome, the result is dryness, which may occur in about 50 percent of patients. This dryness can often lead to cracking and fissuring. This may result in infection, with areas of the skin becoming reddened and itchy. When blood vessels in the skin become inflamed due to white blood cells infiltrating and destroying their walls, the result is vasculitis. This is a rash that resembles red pinpoint spots located over the lower parts of the extremities, particularly the legs. Vasculitis usually occurs over the course of several years following the diagnosis of Sjogren's syndrome. Occasionally the rash may be raised, purple, and painful. This is referred to as palpable purpura. Hypergammaglobulinemic purpura is another type of skin rash; its orange-brown color results from high levels of immunoglobulin circulating in the blood, causing the blood to be thicker than normal and the red blood cells to leak through the superficial blood vessels of the skin. Urticaria or hives can also occur in some patients with Sjogren's syndrome and generally do not itch.

Raynaud's Phenomenon

Another common sign seen in Sjogren's syndrome is Raynaud's phenomenon, which is a three-part response that classically occurs when extremities are exposed to the cold. Generally, the fingers will initially turn white with constriction of blood vessels, then turn blue as a result of pooling of blood in the veins, and finally red when fresh blood reenters the region. Raynaud's phenomenon is seen not only in Sjogren's syndrome but also in a variety of other connective tissue disorders.

Airway Problems

The upper airway, which includes the mouth, nose, and throat, and the lower airway, including the windpipe and lungs, are commonly involved in Sjogren's syndrome. The internal linings of the upper and lower airways, which contain mucus glands, get flooded with lymphocytes (white blood cells) and fail to function properly, leading to dryness. Mucus gland dysfunction may result in laryngotracheobronchitis, which is a chronic inflammatory condition involving the voice box, windpipe, and bronchial tubes. As a result of this inflammation, patients often experience a dry cough. An inability to clear the mucus may result in pneumonia, with fever, chills, and cough being the predominant symptoms of this illness. In addition to pneumonia, patients with Sjogren's syndrome may experience shortness of breath due to a condition known as interstitial pneumonitis. This is an inflammation of the supporting tissue around the alveoli (air sacs) of the lungs. It is important to note that this is a slow process that occurs over years. This type of lung involvement is usually found on X-rays and pulmonary function testing.

Arthritis

Approximately 50 percent of patients with Sjogren's syndrome will experience episodes of arthritis during the course of their disease. These episodes may present as symptoms of arthralgia (joint pain), morning stiffness, or synovitis (intermittent swelling of the joints). X-rays generally tend not to show destructive changes. Some patients with primary Sjogren's syndrome will develop a rheumatoid-like arthritis before the onset of classic Sjogren's symptoms, while true rheumatoid arthritis can also be complicated by the development of dry eye and dry mouth, termed secondary Sjogren's syndrome. In fact, when Henrik Sjogren first described the symptoms of dryness, it was in a group of patients who had an established diagnosis of rheumatoid arthritis. Not surprisingly, the two disorders are sometimes difficult to tell apart.

Gastrointestinal Problems

Sjogren's syndrome may also involve the gastrointestinal tract, leading to symptoms of reflux and dysphagia. Reflux, which is the regurgitation of acid into the esophagus, is thought to result from the inappropriate relaxation of the lower esophageal sphincter. This may be due in part to a dysfunction in the autonomic nervous system, which controls the valve. Lymphocytes infiltrating the nerves may be the cause of this dysfunction. The clinical symptom of reflux is a burning or discomfort in the epigastric area (mid-chest). Excessive acid in the mouth in addition to the existing dryness can also commonly result in mouth sores. Dysphagia (difficulty swallowing) is thought to occur by one of two mechanisms. The first is due to dryness of the pharynx and esophagus, leading to functional inability to swallow. The second mechanism may be due to an actual dysfunction in the movements of the esophagus controlled by the autonomic nervous system. The resultant clinical symptoms include nausea and epigastric pain.

Inflammation of the pancreas has rarely been reported in association with Sjogren's syndrome. Symptoms of this manifestation include nausea, fever, and burning abdominal pain with a radiation to the back. Liver disease has also been reported in some patients with Sjogren's syndrome. Such diseases include autoimmune hepatitis and primary biliary cirrhosis. Patients with these diseases are frequently without symptoms and are diagnosed by routine laboratory testing. With progression of liver disease, some signs and symptoms include pruritis (itching), predominantly of the palms and soles, jaundice (yellowing of skin) and malabsorption of fat.

Kidney Problems

Patients who have kidney involvement present with symptoms of muscle weakness as a result of an electrolyte imbalance known as hypokalemia (low potassium). This electrolyte imbalance often leads to the development of kidney stones, which often cause symptoms of renal colic. Renal colic is recurrent, sharp back pain in the area of the kidney. Interstitial cystitis, which is a nonbacterial (sterile) inflammation of the bladder, can also been seen in Sjogren's syndrome and presents with symptoms such as frequent nighttime urination, suprapubic pain, and dysuria (pain on urination).

Nerve Problems

In rare instances, the nervous system may be involved in Sjogren's syndrome. Symptoms of peripheral neuropathy include numbness, tingling, and burning of the extremities. This may also on rare occasion lead to difficulty with balance. Peripheral neuropathy can also result in symptoms of muscle weakness or abnormal body movements. On physical exam, reflexes may be absent. Cranial neuropathy may also be seen in primary Sjogren's syndrome. One of the most common nerves to be affected is the trigeminal nerve, which supplies sensation to the face and the surface of the eyes as well as to the organs of taste and smell. When this nerve is affected, the result is facial pain or a loss of sensation, taste, or smell. On very rare occasion the central nervous system may also be involved with symptoms resembling those of multiple sclerosis, such as difficulty with speech, balance, blurry vision, movement, and coordination, as well as fine motor skills.

Lymphoma

Lymphoma is another serious disease that can develop in Sjogren's syndrome patients. It manifests as persistent fever, weight loss, and adenopathy of the glands of the neck, armpits, or groin, or swelling and induration of the salivary glands. Benign lymphoproliferative disease (abnormally increased white blood cells in blood or tissue) can often lead to similar symptoms of gland swelling without true lymphoma.

Thyroid Disease

Thyroid disease may also accompany Sjogren's syndrome. The common symptoms of a hypofunctional thyroid include weight gain, cold intolerance, deepening of the voice, coarse hair, excessive fatigue, and depression. Hyperfunctional thyroid disease, known as Graves' disease, can also occur, with symptoms of sweating, palpitations, thinning of the hair, and weight loss. It is important to note that thyroid disease may also occur independently of Sjogren's syndrome.

Vaginal Symptoms

As mentioned previously, dryness is the hallmark of this disease. This dryness can occur on the vaginal surface, thereby decreasing the amount of natural lubrication and resulting in painful intercourse and vaginal burning. Excessive vaginal dryness can also result in various infections.

Depression

Depression has not been studied in Sjogren's syndrome, though it is frequently reported. In a recent survey devised by the Sjogren's Syndrome Foundation, depression was reported in about 29 percent of patients who responded to the survey. This depression is thought to be independent of thyroid disease or fibromyalgia.

Summing Up

It can be seen that Sjogren's syndrome involves more than just dry eye and dry mouth; rather, it is a whole array of symptoms encompassing the entire body. These symptoms may significantly impair a patient's quality of life. However, with prompt recognition and proper treatment, this can be ameliorated.

Abha Gulati, MD

Reza Dana, MD, MPH

7 The Dry Eye

DRY EYE SYNDROME, also called keratoconjunctivitis sicca (KCS), is a component of the dryness (sicca) that characterizes Sjogren's syndrome. The ocular surface consists of the conjunctiva (the mucous membrane covering the outside of the eyeball and the lining of the lids) and the cornea (the central transparent part of the eyeball that allows the light rays to pass through). Dry eye syndrome includes a variety of disorders that affect the ocular surface (both conjunctiva and cornea).

Early diagnosis of dry eye and timely therapy usually help in averting complications, which may be severe; if inadequately treated, it may lead to severe damage to the ocular surface.

The Tear Film

The tear film that covers the surface of the eye consists of three layers: (1) the superficial lipid layer, (2) the middle aqueous layer, and (3) the deep mucin layer (Figure 7.1). The aqueous layer forms the greatest bulk of the tear film and is secreted by the lacrimal (tear-producing) glands (Figure 7.2). The aqueous layer contains water-soluble factors and electrolytes. It helps to wet the conjunctival and corneal surface and causes mechanical flushing of debris and organisms. It acts as a barrier to the entry of toxic substances and microorganisms, and its constituents help inhibit the growth of these microorganisms on the ocular surface. The aqueous layer also contains essential growth factors for the ocular surface cells. See Chapter 4 for more details.

What Changes Occur on the Eye Surface in Dry Eye?

Tears are necessary for the continued health of the ocular surface and for the lubrication required for movement of the lids on the globe. In

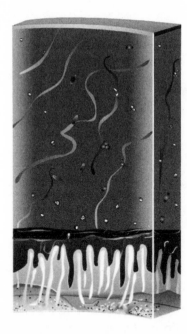

Superficial Lipid Layer
~ 0.1 - 0.2 microns thick

Aqueous Layer
~7-8 microns thick

Adsorbed Mucin Layer
over 1 micron thick

Microvilli of epithelium
extend into and stabilize
mucin layer

Figure 7.1. Diagram showing three layers of the tear film: the superficial lipid layer, the middle aqueous layer, and the deep mucin layer.

the presence of a compromised tear film, the lubricating ability of the tear film is reduced, resulting in greater blink-induced shear force. This blink-induced shear force may be enough to cause changes in the cells of the ocular surface. Moreover, the normal tear film contains essential growth factors that are required for epithelial healing, and deficiency of these factors contributes to impaired healing of the damaged ocular surface in dry eye patients.

The cornea is often more resistant than the conjunctiva to disease in dry eye. The corneal epithelium (the most superficial cell layer) forms a protective barrier between the environment and underlying ocular structures. In moderate to severe dry eye, there is increasing loss of corneal epithelial cells, which are replaced by smaller corneal epithelial cells, or there may be persistent epithelial defects, since the normal healing process is impaired. In severe cases of dry eye, the corneal epithelial defects may enlarge and produce corneal ulcers associated with corneal thinning. These ulcers are initially sterile but may get secondarily infected due to poor healing. In more severe cases, the cornea can thin out con-

Cross-Section of the Eye and Tear Film Producing Structures

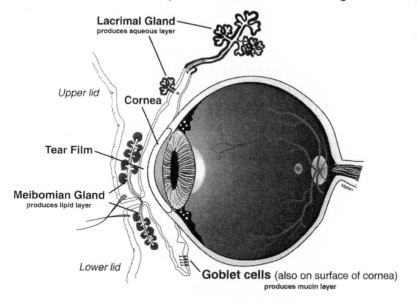

Figure 7.2. Diagram of cross-section of the eye showing tear-film-producing structures.

siderably ("melt") and even perforate, even though the eye often remains white and appears quiet. "Melting" in the context of dry eye is most commonly seen in patients who have rheumatoid arthritis.

How Does a Patient with Dry Eye Present?

The patient's history is extremely important in diagnosing dry eye. Most symptoms in patients with KCS result from an abnormal and inadequately lubricative ocular surface that increases shear forces under the eyelids and diminishes the ability of the ocular surface to respond normally to environmental challenges. Symptoms vary from one patient to another depending on the severity of the dryness, the ability of the diminished tear film to moisten the ocular surface, and the patient's tolerance for ocular discomfort. Patients often use the term *dryness* to describe their condition but will have difficulty defining exactly what it means. The term *discomfort* may be a more accurate summation of all the patient's symptoms. Other frequently encountered symptoms in patients with dry eye are the sensation of a foreign body in the eye or a sandy sensation, burning, and photophobia (difficulty opening eyes in light).

The principal function of the tear film is to maintain a smooth, clear, refractive corneal surface in a hostile external environment. Any adverse effect on the corneal regularity and clarity will interfere with vision. Thus blurred vision may also be one of the initial complaints in a dry eye patient. It is somewhat like looking through a dirty windshield. If the dry eye is due to excessive evaporation, then the patient may feel better by blinking frequently. Patients may also complain of itching, excessive secretion of mucus, heaviness of the eyelids, tight eyelids, and inability to produce tears. Associated inflammation of the surface of the eye may cause pain and redness. Pain may also be due to the filaments (described later) that may form on the surface of the cornea in severe dry eye.

Dry eye patients are highly sensitive to drafts and winds. Often they volunteer information regarding their intolerance to air-conditioning or driving in the car with the windows rolled down. Reading is often difficult for dry eye sufferers. This difficulty probably occurs because the blink frequency decreases during tasks requiring concentration, such as reading or staring at a computer screen. Some patients complain that awakening is the worst part of their day. Sleep (like general anesthesia) decreases tear production. If the eye is already compromised with regard to tear flow, further reduction during sleep may be enough to produce nocturnal symptoms. Smoke is almost universally intolerable to severely tear-deficient patients. Since smoke is actually a suspension of solids in air, the particulate bombardment of the ocular surface produces discomfort. Determining whether symptoms are worse or better indoors or outdoors, at work or at home, will aid in identifying environments that need to be modified to improve a patient's symptoms.

Patients should be asked whether they are able to produce irritant and emotional tears. Inability to cry while peeling onions and when feeling sad or hurt are suggestive of very severe lacrimal gland involvement. Information should be obtained regarding lubricants and medications, including drops as well as ointments. Most patients with KCS improve with topical lubricant therapy. However, excessive use of artificial tears that contain preservatives may worsen the symptoms. Furthermore, any topical medication may be potentially toxic due to the patient's inability to dilute the medication because of a lack of aqueous tear secretion. Some systemic medications such as antiallergics and antidepressants may worsen dry eye symptoms by decreasing tear production.

It is important to determine whether the patient has any other associated systemic signs or symptoms of dryness. Important questions should be directed toward detecting a history of dry mouth. Patients with severe dry mouth will have difficulty swallowing bread or meat without additional fluids. Patients with Sjogren's syndrome and dry mouth are at greater risk of dental and gum disease owing to lack of saliva. Women may experience a noticeable decrease in vaginal secretions, which can lead to sexual dysfunction. A family history should be taken to see whether there is any blood relative with dry eye, Sjogren's syndrome, collagen vascular disease, or other eye diseases.

Clinical Examination

Non-ocular Examination

The facial skin must be inspected for evidence of acne rosacea, which is a condition commonly associated with Meibomian gland dysfunction. Salivary gland enlargement may be seen in patients with Sjogren's syndrome. The thyroid gland should be examined for enlargement and nodules, as thyroid disorders are commonly seen in patients with Sjogren's syndrome.

Ocular Examination

Patients with Sjogren's syndrome may have enlarged lacrimal glands. The size of the lacrimal gland may be evaluated by asking the patient to look down while the upper eyelid is pulled up, but in practice this is not a reliable way of determining lacrimal pathology. In moderate to severe dry eye, the eye appears red due to the presence of inflammation.

A detailed eye examination is performed under magnification using the slit lamp. In dry eye, the conjunctiva and the cornea lose their normal luster. These are seen as a distorted light reflex on the eye surface. Dry eye patients often have excessive tear debris, which probably has two origins. Some of the debris is dead epithelial cells that have fallen off the surface of the cornea, and some are small fibrils of lipid-contaminated mucin that have rolled up and been pushed into the space between the eyeball and the eyelid by the shearing action of the lids.

Another characteristic finding that may be seen in patients with severe dry eye is corneal filaments. Unlike the debris and mucus described above, filaments are actually stuck to the cornea and are not free-floating. It is likely that when the cornea dries to a point that is incompatible with a healthy epithelial layer, some surface cells become desiccated and are shed. As a result, a small pit on the corneal surface appears, to which mucus can attach and serve as a site for adherence of surface epithelial cells, leading to filament formation. Because filaments are anchored to epithelial cells, pulling on them can be very painful. Unfortunately, this is exactly what happens during blinking, with the resultant symptoms not unlike those produced by a foreign body. This form of dry eye is known as filamentary keratitis.

Paralleling the decrease in tear secretion in the lacrimal glands, there is a decrease in certain enzymatic constituents of tears (e.g., lysozyme and lactoferrin, among others), as well as the normal secreted antibodies that protect the eyes from infection. Absence of these protective enzymes and antibodies results in decreased resistance of the eye to infection. Dry eye patients who wear contact lenses are at higher risk of developing contact-lens-associated infections, presumably due to the higher propensity of bacteria to adhere to their contact lenses and ocular surface.

The health of the Meibomian glands must also be assessed. Thick, turbid secretions or the presence of oil or foam suggest Meibomian gland dysfunction. The eyelid margins should be examined for thickening, irregularity, increased blood vessels, and broken and missing eyelashes, which are found in cases of chronic blepharitis (eyelid inflammation).

Tear Secretion Tests

Schirmer Testing

The Schirmer test is the simplest test used for assessing aqueous tear production. Small strips of filter paper, 35 mm long, are used for this test. The strip is placed at the junction of the middle and lateral third of the lower eyelid in both eyes (Figure 7.3). The patient is told to blink normally. Strips are removed after five minutes, and the wetting is recorded in millimeters. The Schirmer test may be done with the eyes open or closed. Less than 6 mm of wetting after five minutes indicates a diagnosis of tear deficiency, although the reliability of this test may be affected by environmental conditions such as temperature or humidity.

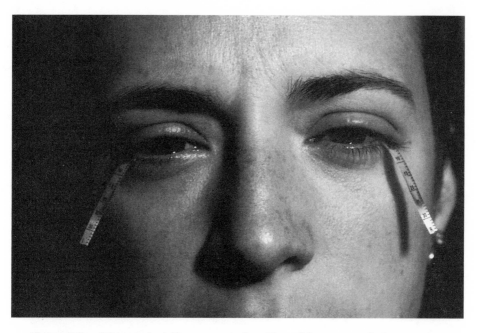

Figure 7.3. Schirmer test. The amount of wetting of the paper strip is a measure of tear secretion.

Rose Bengal Stain

Rose bengal is a red vegetable dye that is used to stain cells that have lost their normal mucin coating. Rose bengal application is a valuable test in the diagnosis of dry eye. It has one disadvantage in that it causes irritation on instillation. The irritation seems to be directly related to the amount of epithelial damage present on the corneal surface and to some extent the size of the drop of dye used. Alternatively, rose bengal strip may be used. A drop of anesthetic may be instilled in the eye before the test to reduce irritation. An alternative to rose bengal is the lissamine green dye test. The dyeing quality of lissamine green is the same as that of rose bengal, and it has the advantage of causing little or no irritation on instillation.

It is important to remember that in dry eye the pattern of the stain, not merely its presence, is important. The stained area corresponds to the exposed surface of the eye. In severe dry eye, the entire cornea tends to stain.

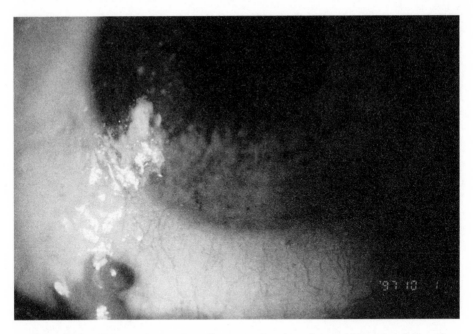

Figure 7.4. Fluorescein staining of cornea showing characteristic of staining of the exposed area of ocular surface in dry eye.

Fluorescein Staining

Fluorescein is a vegetable dye that is used to stain the surface of the eye. It is an orange dye that fluoresces green when excited by blue light. It is typically applied to the eyes with a fluorescein-impregnated strip wetted with a drop of sterile, nonpreserved saline. Fluorescein is able to permeate through a disrupted epithelial layer and diffuse among the intercellular spaces. Thus it gives an indication of the areas on the surface of the eye that have rubbed off due to dryness (Figure 7.4). Fluorescein staining is a standard method used to demonstrate ocular surface damage. Fluorescein instillation is very well tolerated and causes minimal irritation.

Tear Breakup Time

Fluorescein is also useful in staining tears to detect how well the cornea remains continuously covered with a tear film. Tear breakup time (TBUT) tests how well the cornea remains moistened between blinks. After the moistened fluorescein strip is applied to the eye, the patient is asked to blink two or three times to distribute the dye. The test is performed at the slit lamp by asking the patient to stare straight ahead and not blink. Without touching the patient's eyelids, the examiner scans the cornea with the cobalt-blue light of the slit lamp, watching for an area of tear film rupture manifested by a black island within the green sea of fluorescein. The TBUT is the time in seconds between the last blink and the appearance of the first random dry spot. A normal TBUT is considered to be 10 seconds or more, while TBUT is reduced in dry eye.

Laboratory Tests

The following tests for dry eye are most often used in research settings.

Tear Osmolarity

Tear osmolarity tests measure the particle concentration in the tear film. For proper functioning, body fluids normally contain a certain concentration of solutes. Tear osmolarity is a measure of this concentration, which in dry eye patients is hypertonic (elevated osmolarity). Elevated tear osmolarity indicates an imbalance between the rate of tear secretion and the rate of evaporation, in which a decrease in the former or an increase in the latter, or both, is sufficient to disturb the normal balancing mechanisms. Tear hyperosmolarity probably plays an important role in the ocular surface damage in dry eye disease. There are various types of osmometers available for measuring tear osmolarity.

Tear Lysozyme and Lactoferrin

The tear lysozyme test measures lysozyme, which is an enzyme normally present in human tears. Several assay systems are available to determine the level of lysozyme in tears. Normal tear lysozyme levels are between 2 and 4 mg/ml. Patients with Sjogren's syndrome have decreased lysozyme production. Lactoferrin is a stable antibacterial enzyme in tears that can also be measured using multiple tests.

Tear Protein Analysis

Tear protein analysis is based on the rationale that tears from dry eye patients may contain altered protein composition. Tear proteins are measured with the enzyme-linked immunosorbent assay (ELISA), which uses antibodies directed against them. Electrophoresis is a method that can separate various proteins in tears, using their electric gradients. Decreased levels of the goblet-cell-specific mucin MUC5AC have been demonstrated in tears of patients with Sjogren's syndrome.

Conjunctival Impression Cytology

Conjunctival impression cytology is performed using a certain type of filter paper, which is placed on the conjunctiva in order to obtain the impression of the conjunctival epithelium. This test has been used to assay goblet cells in normal subjects and dry eye patients. Reduction in the number of goblet cells is found in dry eye patients.

Conditions That Mimic Dry Eye

Certain eye conditions may be associated with a sensation of dryness. Blepharitis is a common condition that may mimic dry eye. Patients with blepharitis present with symptoms of burning that are worse on awakening, better within an hour or so, and worse again later in the day. There is only modest response to artificial lubricants, but eyelid hygiene done on a regular basis improves symptoms. It is important to emphasize that blepharitis and dry eye can coexist.

In allergic conjunctivitis, symptoms are primarily that of itching. A history of hay fever or atopic dermatitis can be present. Mucin debris may be seen in the tear film. There is usually no rose bengal or fluorescein staining present. It is important to appreciate that allergy and dry eye often coexist. This can be attributed to the fact that in KCS lack of tears and decreased tear turnover may result in an inability to dilute or wash out allergens, increasing the likelihood of allergic conjunctivitis. Conversely, systemic antiallergy medications can exacerbate dryness, and preservatives present in topical antiallergy medicines can also worsen the dry-eye-related eye surface damage.

A variety of conditions in which the surface of the eye may be disrupted may be perceived as dryness. Such conditions include viral infections, contact lens irritation, and medication-induced irritation. The lack of aqueous tear secretion in KCS results in an inability to dilute or wash out substances that the eye comes in contact with, either purposely in the form of topical lubricants or medications, or inadvertently by the application of cosmetics to the face and eyelids. Inability to dilute or wash out potentially toxic substances can cause epithelial and tear film abnormalities. Patients present with symptoms of burning, the sensation of a foreign body, and photophobia, which are present all the time and worsen with continued use of the offending agent.

Social Aspects of Dry Eye

Dry eye is characterized by chronic symptoms of ocular dryness and discomfort that can be debilitating; when severe, they may affect psychological health and the ability to work. Because of the chronic nature of the problem, most patients go through periods of despondency and depression. Ophthalmologists must recognize this part of the illness and actively encourage their patients to continue to pursue their normal activities, remain hopeful, and comply with recommended treatments. The patients should also be asked to stay away from unproven "cures," many of which are touted over the Internet.

8 The Salivary Glands, Ears, Nose, and Larynx

SJOGREN'S SYNDROME IN ITS primary form, also known as the sicca syndrome, is a multisystem disease with a multiplicity of target organs and clinical effects. Understanding the otolaryngologic manifestations of this disease can best be appreciated with a brief introduction to the anatomy of the upper airways and alimentary tract (Figure 8.1).

Anatomy

The lining of the nose, also known as the nasal mucosa, is a moist, fluid-producing organ that is rich in glandular material. In the average adult, the nose and paranasal sinuses secrete about one quart of thin, clear, mucoid fluid a day, which as part of our normal physiology is passed and eventually swallowed. In many disease states, Sjogren's syndrome being a prime example, this physiology is altered, with several manifestations. In the simplest sense, treatment is directed at restoring this mucociliary flow and facilitating the cleansing of the inner tubes and passageways of the head and neck.

A rich network of glandular structures are present on direct examination of the nasal cavity. Laterally in both sides of the nose are the nasal turbinates (passages), which are rich in glands secreting fluid as well as being actively involved in humidification of the airflow and regulating temperature. The secretions often contain various enzymes such as lactoferrin and lysozyme in addition to several types of immunoglobulins, specifically certain subclasses of the IgG molecule as well as the secretory form of the IgA molecule. In a sense, the paranasal sinuses are

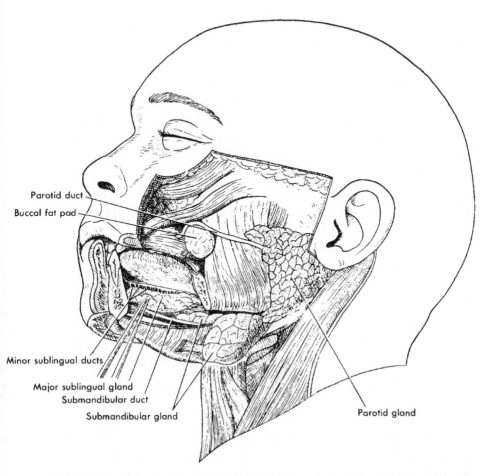

Parotid duct

Buccal fat pad

Minor sublingual ducts

Major sublingual gland

Submandibular duct

Submandibular gland

Parotid gland

Figure 8.1. Salivary glands important in Sjogren's Syndrome. Reprinted from Sichel and DuBrul, *Oral Anatomy*, Mosby, 1975.

a reservoir for producing these secretions as well as acting as a capacitor for the storage of warmth and/or cold as well as humidity. There are probably hundreds of minor salivary glands in the nose as well as the nasopharynx, oral cavity, hypopharynx, and larynx.

As one progresses down the nasopharyngeal tube, one gets to the back of the nose, which in reality is the top of the throat. While the lining here becomes more squamous rather than respiratory in nature, the basic functions of humidification, clearing of particles, and mainte-nance of immunity are still paramount. Additionally, the eustachian tube orifices exit into the nasopharynx, and this is a conduit for draining the middle ear space and by extension the mastoid air cells. Inflammation or disease at this point may have otologic implications. As one continues back down the nasopharynx, the tongue base can be visualized as well as the larynx, where both vocal cords are easily visualized, and one can often see clear, thin fluid coming up from the tracheobronchial tree, which is the lower-airway equivalent of the secretions that begin in the nose and sinuses passages. The hypopharynx also acts as a point or a separate conduit for entering the alimentary tract, that is, the esophagus. A change occurs here, and the lining again is much more squamous and rich in glands such that saliva can be secreted to aid in the early digestion of food particles. Of course, we all know that the oral cavity and the oral tongue are the main inflow point for nutritional support in addition to a bypass mechanism for respiration. A basic understanding of the anatomy therefore is critical to understanding the ear, nose, and throat manifestations of Sjogren's syndrome and by extension its treatments.

Nasal Manifestations

As the autoimmune process within the nasal cavity progresses, one may see the clinical consequences of this destructive process. The de-structive, crust-like pattern is often referred to as atrophic rhinitis. A foul smell, crusts, and even nasal bleeding can be seen. As secretions become thick and occasionally foul-smelling, secondary infection may appear. This can cause further local destruction of the glandular tissue and sometimes even the nasal septum. It is not uncommon to see a perforation of the cartilaginous portion of the nasal septum due to this inflammatory process, with or without secondary bacterial infection.

The paranasal sinuses drain through the various ostia (openings) into the nasal cavity, and with the exception of the sphenoid sinus, they drain from under one of the nasal turbinates. As the inflammatory process proceeds, one may see obstruction of the middle or superior meatus, thus causing secondary outflow problems from the maxillary, ethmoid, and/or frontal sinuses. The narrowest portion of the sinonasal tract in terms of drainage is at the ostiomeatal complex, which is anatomically close to the middle meatus. Even mild local inflammation can cause sinus infections. Symptoms include pain, headache, and occasional fever, in addition to the atrophic symptoms. Many patients will complain of anosmia (loss of smell) and a sense of fullness inside the nose. Secondary infections of the paranasal sinuses need to be treated medically.

My personal bias in treating Sjogren's of the nose and sinus tract revolves around humidification and replacement of what is lost. Specifically, water in all its forms is critical for reversing the atrophic/inflammatory destruction and for allowing the passage of thick, crusty material down into the oral cavity so that it can eventually be swallowed or spit out through the mouth. The overriding principle here is one of humidification using clean, balanced saline solutions. There are various brands of over-the-counter saline sprays, and I have no preference for any particular one. The critical point here is constant and prophylactic humidification and saline replacement. Recently, a longer-acting form of nasal lubricant is available that is glycol-based (trade name Rhinaris). It comes both as a mist and as a gel, with the latter being particularly useful for longer-term lubrication and hydration, particularly while sleeping. The use of topical intranasal steroids is often suggested, although its efficacy has yet to be clearly demonstrated.

Additionally, some people with severe crusting need to irrigate with a WaterPik, and various nasal attachments exist that help to facilitate nasal hygiene. Other devices such as a Netti Pot may have value, as do hot, steamy showers. For all patients with Sjogren's syndrome, the use of concurrent medications that can facilitate dryness needs to be avoided; this particularly is important with respect to antihistamines and systemic decongestants.

How Is the Ear Affected in Sjogren's?

Hearing loss as a result of Sjogren's disease is uncommon but does occur. Some autoimmune diseases have clearly been linked with a sensorineural (nerve-type) deafness; however, this does not appear to be the case here. There are patients, however, who occasionally complain of either tinnitus, hearing loss, or otalgia in small degrees; this can be as high as one-quarter of all patients. Because the middle-ear fluid needs to drain into the back of the nose through the eustachian tube orifice, disease with severe inflammation in the nasal cavity could potentially block the eustachian tube or cause an inflammatory condition resulting in a conductive hearing loss. Fortunately, this is easily treated with either ventilating tubes, amplification devices, or local hygiene. Sometimes, increased doses of immunosuppressives or steroids may have value.

How Is the Mouth Affected in Sjogren's?
See Chapter 9.

How Is the Larynx Affected in Sjogren's?
The larynx or voice box is involved in protecting the airway from foreign bodies and promoting good airflow into the tracheobronchial tree. It is also involved in diverting food to the alimentary tract (esophagus), and it is the most critical organ in terms of our ability to phonate. Laryngeal disorders in Sjogren's are often manifested by coughing and occasionally hoarseness. Voice changes may be present, as the glands below the vocal cords and the trachea are also affected in addition to the minor salivary glands from above. Patients infrequently develop respiratory symptoms attributable to Sjogren's; however, professional singers or people who use their voice frequently during the day are at increased risk for chronic laryngitis and its sequelae. Inspissation (thickening) of mucus and other secretions can cause a foul smell and occasionally a sense of blockage in one's airway. As in treating disease in the mouth, vigorous oral hydration is the primary treatment in addition to systemic immune system modulation with either steroids or glandular stimulation with drugs such as cevimeline and pilocarpine. Other treatments include voice rest and occasionally guaifenesin-containing products to help thin mucus, not only in the nasal tract but also in the tracheobronchial tree.

Summing Up
The otolaryngologic (ear, nose, and throat) manifestations of Sjogren's disease are significant and varied. It is critical to remind patients and their physicians to limit drugs that can dry the mucous membranes

within the upper airways. Antihistamines and decongestants are but two of the medications that have these effects. Oral hydration and replacement with artificial saliva have value, as does replacing sinonasal secretions with saline or glycol-based nose sprays. Guaifenesin is useful in helping the larynx to clear itself.

Ava J. Wu, DDS

Troy E. Daniels, DDS, MS

9 The Dry Mouth: A Dental Perspective On Sjogren's

SOMETIMES A DENTIST IS the first to diagnose Sjogren's. Dry mouth is a common complaint that can have many causes. This symptom is often referred to as xerostomia. It is usually caused by a decrease in the amount and quality of saliva, but because it is a subjective perception, abnormalities in salivary function may not be observed in all patients with this complaint. Almost all Sjogren's syndrome patients experience some degree of dry mouth.

Causes of Dry Mouth

The most common cause of dry mouth is from the use of certain types of drugs. Hundreds of drugs in several categories are known to cause dry mouth as a side effect (Table 9.1). Clinical experience suggests also that interactions may occur between different drugs not usually associated with dry mouth, causing that symptom. In most cases, the drugs causing dry mouth do so through their effect on nerves that regulate salivary function.

Sjogren's syndrome is a systemic autoimmune disease that causes dry mouth by way of lymphocytes (a type of white blood cell) infiltrating the salivary glands. These infiltrating cells replace the normal salivary gland cells that produce the secretion (acinar cells) and affect the function of duct cells that convey the secretion to the mouth. Recent research also shows that Sjogren's patients may produce an antibody in their

TABLE 9.1   DRUGS COMMONLY ASSOCIATED WITH DRY MOUTH*

Antianxiety: alprazolam
Antihypertensive: clonidine; methyldopa
Antidepressant: amitriptyline (+++);** buproprion (0); citalopram (0/+);
   doxepin (++); fluoxetine (0/+); imipramine (++); mirtazapine (0); nefazodone
   (0/+); nortriptyline (++); paroxetine (+); sertraline (0); venlafaxine (0/+)
Antihistamine/antiemetic: brompheniramine (++); cetirizine (0/+);
   chlorpheniramine (++); diphenhydramine (+++); hydroxyzine (++);
   loratadine (0/+); perchlorperazine (++); promethazine (++++)
Antipsychotic: chlorpromazine (++); clozapine (+++); fluphenazine (+);
   haloperidol (0/+); loxapine (+); molindone (+); olanzapine (+); quetiapine (+);
   risperidone (0/+); thioridazine (+++); thiothixene (+); trifluoperazine (+);
   ziprasidone (0/+)
Anti-Parkinson's: benztropine; selegiline; trihexyphenidyl
Antiacne: isotretinoin
Decongestant: pseudoephedrine
Bronchodilator: ipratropium; albuterol
Muscle relaxant: cyclobenzaprine

Rating of anticholinergic (drying) effects: 0 none; 0/+ very low; + low; ++
moderate; +++ high
*For consistency and clarity, all drugs are listed by their generic names, alpha-
betically. There are hundreds of drugs associated with dry mouth, but with most
of them, the symptom is generally mild, occurs in a small minority of patients taking
the drug, or the drug is not prescribed for chronic use. This list includes the categories of drugs that most commonly cause significant dry mouth, but it is not all
inclusive. When questions arise, patients should consult with their physician or a
reliable drug information source.
Source: Anderson PO, Knoben JE, Troutman WG, *Handbook of Clinical Drug
Data*, 10th ed. McGraw-Hill, 2002.

bloodstream that can affect the nerves regulating salivary function. The
onset of dry mouth symptoms in patients with Sjogren's is very gradual,
and most patients cannot determine exactly when it began. It may progress gradually until little or no saliva is produced, but more commonly,
patients' symptoms and salivary dysfunction progress to some interme-
diate point and do not progress further.

As mentioned previously, the use of prescription drugs can play a
significant role in causing or exacerbating the sensation of dry mouth.
Accordingly, patients with Sjogren's must review with their physicians
any prescription drugs they are taking, to ensure that those drugs are
not increasing their dry mouth. Often, there are alternative and equivalent drugs available that are not as drying (Table 9.1).

Dry mouth can also be caused by other chronic diseases such as

---

TABLE 9.2   CAUSES OF DRY MOUTH

Temporary dry mouth

- Effects of short-term drug use (*e.g.,* antihistamines)
- Virus infections* (*e.g.,* mumps)
- Dehydration (*e.g.,* heat or injury)
- Psychogenic conditions (*e.g.,* anxiety)

Chronic dry mouth

- Effects of chronically administered drugs (see Table 9.1)
- Chronic diseases
  - Sjogren's syndrome*
  - Sarcoidosis*
  - HIV* or hepatitis C infection
  - Depression
  - Diabetes mellitus, uncontrolled
  - Amyloidosis (primary or secondary)
  - Central nervous system diseases
  - Rarely, absent or malformed glands
- Other effects of treatment
- Therapeutic radiation to the head and neck
- Graft-versus-host disease (following bone marrow transplantation)

---

*These conditions may also cause major salivary gland enlargement

---

sarcoidosis, HIV or hepatitis C infection, uncontrolled diabetes, or depression. Previous medical treatments such as radiation therapy to the head and neck, bone marrow transplantation (graft-versus-host disease), or chemotherapy for treating malignancies can damage the salivary glands and cause decreased salivation (Table 9.2). The effects of such treatment can be either temporary or permanent, depending on the type and intensity of treatment.

Temporary symptoms of dry mouth, such as when taking over-the-counter drugs for treating cold symptoms, are not important. However, if dry mouth and diminished salivation continues for many weeks or months, regardless of the cause, detrimental changes will begin to occur to the teeth and oral function.

The Functions of Saliva

Saliva is an essential body fluid whose critical role in oral comfort and function is seldom appreciated until there is not enough of it. It is created by three pairs of major salivary glands, the parotid, submandibular, and sublingual glands, and by hundreds of minor glands located in many areas of the mouth. All of these glands can be affected by Sjogren's. Saliva is composed mostly of water but includes small amounts of many substances that have important roles in protecting and preserving the teeth, oral soft tissues, and oral function. These roles include:

- *Protecting, lubricating and cleansing the oral mucosa.* Saliva coats tissues of the mouth and ingested food allowing the food to pass smoothly over the teeth and oral soft tissue. This coating facilitates chewing and swallowing and acts as a barrier to irritating and harmful substances contained in food. The salivary coating inside the mouth also facilitates speech.

- *Protecting against dental caries (decay).* As discussed below, dental caries results from the exposure of teeth to acid produced by adhering bacterial plaques. Saliva contains several chemical systems, called buffers, that can neutralize the acidity of foods and beverages to maintain a neutral pH (a measure of the chemical balance between acidic and alkaline). Saliva also contains reservoirs of calcium and phosphate ions that replenish those elements as they are gradually lost from teeth. Secretory IgA is a unique antibody found in saliva that can coat many oral bacteria, interfering with their ability to adhere to teeth.

- *Protecting against infection by bacteria, yeasts, and viruses.* There are several protein components in saliva (for example, lactoferrin, peroxidase, histatins, and secretory leukocyte protease) that have antibacterial, antifungal, and antiviral properties.

- *Aiding digestion and taste.* Initial stages of digestion occur in the mouth by way of enzymes contained in saliva. Taste buds, which are located in the mouth, can only respond to dissolved substances; saliva enhances the sense of taste by both dissolving and digesting solid foods. The solvent and digestive roles of saliva allow the taste buds to convey food flavors that enhance enjoyment of any meal.

Oral Problems Caused by Chronic Dry Mouth

Clearly, saliva is important for the quality of life. Progressive loss of saliva production correspondingly erodes the beneficial and protective effects of saliva listed above. The most severely affected patients with

Sjogren's do not produce measurable amounts of saliva, but most patients retain residual salivary gland function, ranging from a small amount to almost normal.

Dry Mouth Symptoms

The critical damage threshold for decreased salivary function has not yet been defined. It has been shown, however, that the sensation of dry mouth does not occur for an individual until saliva production drops to approximately one-half that person's baseline value. The feeling of intraoral dryness associated with Sjogren's often develops over a period of months or years. Sudden onset of oral dryness is rare in Sjogren's. Occasionally, an individual is not aware of being dry until asked if he or she can swallow a cracker without water. The severity of oral dryness in patients with Sjogren's may fluctuate, but it usually does not include periods of time during the day where their mouth feels normal.

Normally, little saliva is produced during sleep, so it is common for all individuals to feel some oral dryness in the morning or on awakening during the night. This symptom may be more severe for patients with Sjogren's and should be managed with small amounts of a commercial saliva substitute or a secretogogue, instead of water, to avoid sleep disruption caused by the urge to urinate.

Dental Caries

The process of tooth decay is caused by interactions between several types of bacteria commonly found in the mouth and particular sugars present in the diet of most individuals. These bacteria form plaques, coating the teeth so rapidly that they can be seen by the unaided eye after only a day or two without tooth brushing. If an individual's diet includes sucrose (common table sugar) or other sugars that can be metabolized by these bacteria, the organisms grow rapidly in number and produce increasing amounts of acid from their metabolism of the sugar. The acid in turn progressively dissolves the mineral content of the teeth (called decalcification), to which the organisms adhere.

For individuals who have a deficient amount of saliva, dental caries progresses more rapidly and in different dental locations, even in those with good oral hygiene. The pattern of dry mouth caries is distinctive. Caries is located on the necks of teeth near the gum line, the cusp tips of back teeth, or the biting edges of front teeth. This is in contrast to dental caries in individuals with normal saliva but inadequate oral hygiene, where caries occur between teeth and in pits and fissures on the chewing surfaces of back teeth. In addition, dry mouth patients often exhibit recurrent caries along the margins of existing dental restorations, ultimately causing the restorations to fail.

Insufficient saliva contributes to increased dental decay in several ways: (1) a decreased ability to buffer acids that are ingested or produced by bacteria adhering to teeth, (2) an insufficient reservoir of calcium and phosphate ions to replenish that naturally lost from teeth, (3) a reduction of antimicrobial proteins, and (4) reduced oral cleansing from lower salivary flow.

Dental caries usually causes no symptoms until it penetrates through the surface enamel of the tooth into the dentin. Dental enamel is very dense and composed almost entirely of nonorganic material, like ivory, while dentin is like bone, with many organic components, including nerves. After caries enters the dentin, that tooth usually becomes sensitive to heat or cold. If untreated, caries can progress through the dentin into the pulp, where the bacteria infect the dental pulp, causing increased pain (pulpitis). From the pulp, invading bacteria can expand into the bone adjacent to the root tip, causing a painful abscess. Early dental caries appears as a flat, whitish spot on a tooth's surface (decalcification). As the process continues, there is progressive loss of tooth structure, and a cavity appears that can be tan to black in color.

Fungal Infection

About one-third of patients with chronic salivary deficiency have symptoms of burning in their tongue or elsewhere in their mouth and/ or intolerance to acidic or spicy foods. These symptoms are usually caused by localized infection of the lining the mouth (stomatopyrosis) by different species of the fungus candida. This organism is often a normal inhabitant of the oral flora, but in susceptible patients with deficient saliva, candida can proliferate and cause those symptoms. Where this has occurred, the tongue appears red, loses its normal carpet-like surface texture, and may develop surface grooves. Other affected areas develop well-defined or diffuse red areas caused by thinning of the mucosa (called atrophy). These intraoral changes are often associated with redness or crusting at the corners of the lips, called angular cheilitis. This combination of clinical features is called erythematous candidiasis. Effective treatment with antifungal drugs will lead to complete restoration of the mucosal changes and elimination of the symptoms, despite ongoing salivary deficiency. However, in susceptible patients, this condition often recurs, necessitating retreatment, which can be repeated as often as necessary.

Oral Functional Problems

It is common for patients with Sjogren's to have difficulty swallowing dry foods because they have insufficient saliva to adequately moisten the bolus of food. They may also have difficulty speaking because the tongue and lips have insufficient salivary lubrication. As noted in Chapter 15, these can be overcome by frequent sips of water and/or use of secretogogues. Sjogren's patients wearing complete dentures often experience progressive difficulty because deficient oral lubrication may cause the tongue to continually move the lower denture. Where it is possible to do so, implants surgically imbedded within the lower jaw may provide a means to stabilize the lower denture.

Periodontal Disease

It is often argued that in Sjogren's increased amounts of bacterial plaque will develop on teeth, which should cause greater gum inflammation (gingivitis). However, most research papers that have addressed the question of whether patients with Sjogren's have more severe gum disease than the general population have found no difference between the groups. Perhaps patients with Sjogren's are more aware of the beneficial effect of careful hygiene and have better oral hygiene than the general population, which could play a role in investigators' inability to find more severe periodontal disease in Sjogren's patients.

Halitosis (Bad Breath)

Halitosis can occur when there is an overgrowth of certain types of odor-causing bacteria. These bacteria can be the result of active dental caries or periodontal disease, inadequate oral hygiene, or deficient saliva such as in Sjogren's. This problem is managed by appropriate dental or periodontal treatment to eradicate underlying disease along with regular and careful oral hygiene.

Salivary Gland Enlargement

Salivary gland enlargement or swelling occurs in about one-third of patients with Sjogren's, while the majority of Sjogren's patients never experience this change. The enlargement is gradual in onset and without symptoms or with only mild symptoms of discomfort. It can slowly regress and recur over periods of many months or become chronic. In rare cases of Sjogren's, these enlargements can transform into a malignant condition, usually lymphoma. In patients experiencing this enlargement, it may be appropriate to consider other causes of the enlargement by way of magnetic resonance imaging, fine-needle aspiration for cytology, or salivary gland biopsy.

Diagnostic Testing of Dry Mouth

Dry mouth from Sjogren's and other causes is diagnosed by both dentists and physicians with a combination of methods.

Symptoms and Follow-up Questions

The range of symptoms experienced by patients with Sjogren's is discussed in the section above. In patients complaining of dry mouth, it is also helpful to know if their mouth feels dry while eating, if they need water for swallowing solid foods, or if they need water to chew and swallow dry foods. Positive responses to these questions have a significant association with decreased saliva production.

Salivary and Oral Examination

In examining patients suspected of having Sjogren's, the major salivary glands should be palpated for evidence of tenderness, changes in consistency, or enlargement. Saliva expressed from the major salivary ducts intraorally should be visually assessed for its clarity, viscosity, and wetting ability. The oral mucosa should be assessed for its lubricity (normally wet and slippery versus dry and sticky) and its color. The extent and pattern of dental caries must be noted, as described in the section above.

Salivary Flow Rate Measurement (Sialometry)

Salivary gland function is most easily assessed by collecting saliva over a specified period of time. The collection can be made from separate glands, such as the parotid, using special collectors, or of whole saliva collected simply by expectoration (spitting). These collections can be made under conditions that stimulate salivary secretion (for example, while chewing or tasting) or without stimulation, yielding quite different results with different diagnostic potential. These are all painless, non-invasive tests that are useful to assess the presence and severity of salivary dysfunction and to monitor patients' disease progress over time and the effects of treatment. There is no universally accepted measure that defines abnormal salivary function, but an unstimulated whole salivary flow rate of less than 1 ml/10 minutes is widely accepted as a threshold of abnormal function. Reductions in salivary flow rate are caused by many different conditions, and none are diagnostically specific.

Scintigraphy

This test measures the rate at which a small amount of injected radioactive material is taken up from the blood into the salivary glands and secreted into the mouth. It is another method to measure salivary gland function that may be helpful for evaluating individuals with severe salivary dysfunction.

Sialography

This technique uses a liquid radiographic contrast medium injected into a salivary duct followed by X-ray images of that gland to exhibit its ductal structure. The technique is useful to explore duct obstructions and distinguish between chronic inflammatory changes and neoplasms, but it is limited in its ability to provide diagnostically specific information about Sjogren's. Sialography in patients with significant salivary hypofunction must be done with water-based contrast media to avoid the risk of chronic foreign body reaction from use of oil-based media.

Ultrasound and Magnetic Resonance Imaging (MRI)

These are non-invasive imaging techniques that can examine salivary glands for structural changes. Ultrasound examination may be helpful in identifying vascular or cystic lesions in salivary glands. MRI is an excellent technique for imaging masses in salivary glands, particularly as part of presurgical evaluation. There have been only a few studies examining these techniques in the context of Sjogren's. The possibility of diagnostic applications for Sjogren's have been suggested, but evidence of their usefulness is inconclusive at this time.

Sialochemistry

These techniques examine saliva for the presence and amount of particular substances. Sialochemistry has been applied to compare saliva samples from normal individuals to those from Sjogren's patients with the hope of identifying differences that can be used as diagnostic criteria for Sjogren's. Differences between normal and Sjogren's saliva have been identified, but many of those differences are caused by reduced salivary function, not specifically by Sjogren's.

Minor Salivary Gland Biopsy

This test, also commonly referred to as a lip biopsy, is currently considered the gold standard for diagnosing the salivary component of Sjogren's. Using local anesthesia, a small, shallow incision is made on the inner surface of the lower lip to directly visualize and remove at least four of these small glands. There are hundreds of these minor salivary glands located throughout the mouth, which are between 1/16 and 1/8 inch (1 and 3 mm) in diameter. This technique is preferable to the punch biopsy technique, which is a blind procedure; it usually does not yield a sufficient sample of minor glands and may endanger sensory nerves in the area. A pathologist then examines the glands for the presence of changes characteristic of the salivary component of Sjogren's, or occasionally of other diseases.

Summing Up

The symptom of dry mouth can be the result of diverse causes. It is important to determine if it is the result of decreased salivary function from a disease such as Sjogren's, from the chronic use of a drug known to cause dry mouth, or from a combination of both. With this knowledge, preventive measures can be taken to minimize the effects of this potentially important physiological change.

Fotini C. Soliotis, MD

Stuart S. Kassan, MD

Haralampos Moutsopoulos, MD

10 The Internal Organs in Sjogren's

IN SJOGREN'S SYNDROME the immune system primarily targets the salivary and lacrimal glands. However, less commonly the same immune process can also affect the major organs of the body, such as the lungs, the heart, the gut, the liver, the kidney, and the nervous system. Major organ disease is only seen in one-third of primary Sjogren's patients and can be divided into two categories depending on whether it manifests itself early (that is, together with the symptoms of dry eye and dry mouth) or later on, sometimes years after the diagnosis of Sjogren's has been made.

Manifestations of lung and liver disease as well as one type of kidney disease (interstitial nephritis) occur early, around the time of diagnosis of Sjogren's, and are unlikely to occur later on. These diseases are characterized by a common immune process: an infiltration of the affected organ by a group of white cells called lymphocytes.

On the other hand, the less common type of kidney disease, glomerulonephritis, and the involvement of the peripheral nerves often occur later in the disease process and are not present at the time of diagnosis of Sjogren's. These two diseases are also characterized by a common immune process: inflammation of blood vessels, known as vasculitis, caused by the deposition of immune complexes (structures made up of antibodies) on the vessel walls.

Although disease of the major body organs is rarely severe or life-threatening in Sjogren's, it should nevertheless be diagnosed promptly so that effective treatment is given. This is one of the reasons why Sjogren's patients should be monitored by their physician on a regular basis.

The Respiratory Tract

The entire respiratory tract may be affected in Sjogren's. Starting from the nose, thinning of the mucous membrane of the nose, or atrophic rhinitis, can occur, giving rise to nasal dryness. Moving down the airway, the voice box (larynx), windpipe (trachea), and bronchial tubes can become inflamed; this is known as laryngotracheobronchitis. The main symptoms of this condition are hoarseness of the voice, dry cough, wheezing and shortness of breath.

Because there is less mucus produced in the airway, Sjogren's patients have difficulty clearing foreign material that has been inhaled into the respiratory tract. This can also contribute to the chronic inflammation of the bronchi and can predispose the patient to bacterial infections. Also, mucus can become stuck in the small bronchi, blocking the ventilation of a small segment of the lung. This can lead to the collapse of that lung segment (known as atelectasis).

Inflammation of the trachea and bronchi (tracheobronchitis) can be diagnosed by performing breathing tests known as pulmonary function tests. The patient blows into a tube connected to a machine that measures the flow of air in the bronchi. In this way the reduced flow of air in the bronchial tubes can be detected. In tracheobronchitis a standard chest X-ray can be normal.

The use of room humidifiers can be of help in relieving the symptoms of mild tracheobronchitis. Also, prescribed nebulizers, which can deliver tiny water droplets into the small airways, may be useful. If the patient is wheezing or if the pulmonary function tests confirm blockage of airflow in the bronchi, then inhalers containing medications that dilate the bronchi can be prescribed. However, these are only partially effective, as they cannot clear the mucus blocking the bronchi. In this respect, drugs that break down mucus (mucolytics) may be of some benefit.

The lung itself can also become inflamed in Sjogren's (interstitial lung disease, ILD). As the bronchi branch out they end up in small air sacs known as the alveoli, where carbon dioxide is exchanged for oxygen. Around the alveoli there is supporting tissue known as the interstitium. This contains small blood vessels that take up the oxygen from the alveoli. If there is inflammation and scarring within the interstitium, then less oxygen can enter the blood within the lungs.

The symptoms of interstitial lung disease vary depending on the severity of the disease. In the early stages patients may have no symptoms or may complain of a dry cough and mild shortness of breath on exertion. In the late stages of severe ILD, which is rare, patients may have disabling breathlessness on exertion.

The chest X-ray may show a lacy or honeycomb type of shadowing within the lungs. Pulmonary function tests show impairment of gas transfer from the alveoli into the blood vessels and a reduced volume of air in the lungs. High-resolution computed tomography scans (HRCT) of the lungs are very useful in confirming the diagnosis. When looking at HRCT films, areas of inflammation appear as patches of white "ground glass" within the dark lungs. However, other lung conditions can mimic interstitial lung disease associated with Sjogren's, and therefore further investigations are sometimes necessary in order to confirm the diagnosis. In a procedure known as bronchoscopy, a tube can be inserted from the nose inside the lungs with the patient awake. Then a sample of bronchial secretions can be obtained and examined under the microscope. In ILD associated with Sjogren's, fluid from bronchial secretions typically contains numerous lymphocytes, which are cells involved in inflammation. Sometimes a lung biopsy, done either during bronchoscopy or through a chest incision under local anesthetic (open-lung biopsy), is needed to make the diagnosis. The standard treatment for ILD is corticosteroids given either by mouth or intravenously. Depending on the response and on the severity of the disease, it may also be necessary to add other immunosuppressive drugs such as azathioprine or cyclophosphamide. If treated early, ILD does not cause any long-term disability.

Inflammation of the lining around the lung (pleurisy) can occur in Sjogren's. This condition is usually seen in patients with secondary Sjogren's syndrome and particularly in those suffering from systemic lupus erythematosus or rheumatoid arthritis. Pleurisy usually causes chest pain on breathing. Fluid can sometimes accumulate in the pleural space (pleural effusion) causing shortness of breath. Pleurisy is treated with non-steroidal anti-inflammatory drugs or corticosteroids. Also, drainage of the pleural effusion may sometimes be necessary.

Very rarely Sjogren's patients develop an abnormally high pressure in the pulmonary arteries, the vessels that carry blood from the heart to the lungs. This is known as pulmonary hypertension. The main symptom of pulmonary hypertension is shortness of breath on exertion. In Sjogren's, pulmonary hypertension can develop in isolation or as a result of ILD and lung scarring (fibrosis). Pulmonary hypertension can be diagnosed on a routine cardiac echocardiogram. To obtain an accurate measurement of the pulmonary artery pressure, the patient undergoes cardiac catheterization. Under local anesthetic, a thin wire is guided from the artery in the leg into the main aorta and then into the right side of the heart so that measurements of pressure can be taken. If left untreated, severe pulmonary hypertension can cause heart failure. Treatment of any underlying interstitial lung disease can help improve the degree of pulmonary hypertension. The use of intravenous epoprostenol and anticoagulants has greatly improved the life expectancy of patients with severe pulmonary hypertension. More recently a new oral drug, bosentan, has also been shown to be an effective treatment.

Kidneys

The kidneys remove waste products from the blood and form urine. The most common kidney problem in patients with Sjogren's syndrome is inflammation of the tissue around the kidney filters, known as interstitial nephritis. Interstitial nephritis is found early in the disease and has a benign course. It generally causes mild deterioration in kidney function, manifested as a mild elevation in the plasma creatinine concentration. This usually requires no treatment. Progression to end-stage renal disease is a rare event. When there is progressive deterioration of kidney function in a patient with Sjogren's syndrome, a kidney biopsy is often done. This involves taking a small piece of kidney tissue with a needle while the patient is awake, under local anesthetic. The tissue is examined under the microscope, and if the diagnosis of interstitial nephritis is made, a course of corticosteroids is given as treatment. Kidney function usually improves within a few weeks unless irreversible scarring in the kidneys has already occurred.

Interstitial nephritis can cause abnormalities in the kidney tubules, which are part of the kidney filtering mechanism. One such abnormality is renal tubular acidosis (RTA). In RTA the kidney tubules are unable to excrete acid in the urine. This can occur in up to 25 percent of patients with Sjogren's syndrome. As a result, the urine becomes more alkaline (high urine pH) and the blood becomes more acidic (low blood pH). This can lead to low levels of potassium in the blood and can give rise to kidney stones. Patients with RTA usually have no symptoms. Rarely, when the blood potassium level is very low, muscle weakness or even paralysis can occur. Also, recurrent pain in the loin area, caused by kidney stones, can sometimes be the presenting symptom. The treatment of RTA depends on its severity. If the potassium level is very low, then the patient is given potassium supplements to take in the form of tablets. Alkaline agents (sodium bicarbonate) are given to correct the acidity of the blood so as to prevent the formation of renal stones.

Another rare abnormality of the renal tubules in Sjogren's syndrome is nephrogenic diabetes insipidus. In this condition the renal tubules become insensitive to the effects of anti-diuretic hormone and as a result cannot concentrate the urine. Patients with nephrogenic diabetes insipidus complain of thirst and of passing large amounts of urine frequently. The diagnosis is suspected if the urine remains dilute when the patient is deprived of water (when a normal person becomes dehydrated the kidneys try to save water by concentrating the urine). Nephrogenic diabetes insipidus can be treated by a number of means, including the use of diuretics, non-steroidal anti-inflammatory drugs, and a low-salt, low-protein diet.

The glomeruli, which also form part of the kidney filtering mechanism, are rarely affected in Sjogren's syndrome. Antibodies produced by the immune system become deposited on the glomeruli and cause inflammation (glomerulonephritis). As a result, the function of the kidneys deteriorates. This can be picked up on routine testing of a sample of urine and by looking at the blood tests and observing a deterioration of kidney function. Symptoms include high blood pressure and leg swelling due to water retention (edema). Glomerulonephritis is rare in patients with Sjogren's and occurs mainly in those patients who also have other overlapping conditions such as systemic lupus erythematosus, cryoglobulinemia (a condition whereby protein complexes circulating in the blood become deposited during cold weather), and vasculitis (inflammation of blood vessels). If left untreated, glomerulonephritis may lead to severe kidney failure. Therefore in a patient with suspected glomerulonephritis a kidney biopsy should be performed to confirm the diagnosis and assess the severity of the kidney disease. Treatment is then given in the form of corticosteroids as well as other immunosuppressive drugs (cyclophosphamide).

Inflammation of the bladder, known as interstitial cystitis, can occur in patients with Sjogren's. The symptoms are frequent urination and pain in the lower abdomen over the bladder area.

The Gastrointestinal Tract

In Sjogren's the exocrine glands of the gastrointestinal tract can also be affected. The cells lining the esophagus produce less mucus, and the esophagus becomes dry like the mouth. This can lead to difficulty in swallowing. Difficulty in swallowing can also be caused by abnormal contractions of the esophagus or by a lack of the normal contractions that move the food down the esophagus to the stomach. This condition, which can affect up to one-third of patients with Sjogren's, is known as esophageal dysmotility.

The diagnosis of dysmotility is made by measuring the pressure inside the wall of the esophagus during swallowing (manometry). When the wall of the esophagus contracts abnormally, treatment is aimed at relaxing the smooth muscle of the esophagus. Nitroglycerin and calcium channel blockers may be helpful.

On the other hand, when the muscle tone in the wall of the esophagus is reduced, gastric juice moves up the esophagus, producing a burning sensation behind the breastbone (heartburn) and chest pain. This is known as gastro-esophageal reflux. Prolonged reflux of acid results in chronic irritation of the esophagus (esophagitis). Mild reflux can be treated by the use of antacids. Antacids form a "raft" that floats on the surface of the stomach contents to reduce reflux and protect the lining of the esophagus. Severe gastro-esophageal reflux and esophagitis are best treated by the use of drugs that reduce acid production by the stomach. These include H_2-receptor antagonists (ranitidine) and proton pump inhibitors (omeprazole).

However, a proportion of patients with Sjogren's have reduced acid secretion by the stomach. This is a result of long-standing inflammation that destroys the cells that produce acid (chronic atrophic gastritis), an immune process similar to the one that destroys the salivary glands. Atrophic gastritis can cause indigestion (dyspepsia) and pain over the upper part of the abdomen. Diagnosis is made by endoscopy. This is performed by a gastroenterologist with the patient awake but slightly sedated. The stomach is visualized by inserting an elastic tube with a camera at its end (fiber-optic endoscope) inside the stomach. A biopsy is often taken to confirm the diagnosis. Unfortunately, once the acid-producing cells of the stomach are damaged, it is often too late to give any treatment.

However, other conditions associated with atrophic gastritis can be prevented. Destruction of the cells that produce acid in the stomach can prevent absorption of vitamin B_{12}, important in the production of red blood cells. Its deficiency can result in a form of anemia known as pernicious anemia. Pernicious anemia can be diagnosed by a simple blood test and can be successfully treated by B_{12} injections (see Chapter 16).

In Sjogren's, involvement of other exocrine glands such as the pancreas can sometimes occur. Most of the time this does not cause any symptoms. However, in some cases the pancreas cannot secrete its digestive enzymes, and then the symptoms are diarrhea and steatorrhea (floating, fatty stools). Pancreatic enzyme insufficiency can be treated by the regular administration of oral pancreatic enzymes.

Acute inflammation of the pancreas, known as pancreatitis, has been rarely described in Sjogren's patients. It presents with abdominal pain, nausea, and vomiting. Laboratory tests show elevation of amylase, an enzyme measured in the serum. Amylase is produced by the salivary glands as well as by the pancreas. A quarter of patients with Sjogren's may have a raised serum amylase due to salivary gland inflammation rather than due to acute pancreatitis.

The Liver

In studies of Sjogren's patients, approximately 6 percent are found to have autoimmune liver disease. The main two conditions associated with Sjogren's are chronic active hepatitis and primary biliary cirrhosis.

Primary biliary cirrhosis (PBC) is a chronic disease that affects mainly middle-aged women. It is caused by inflammation around the channels that transport bile from the liver into the intestine, the bile ducts. As a result, these ducts become blocked, and bile builds up in the liver and spills into the blood. In the late stages of the disease the liver becomes scarred. This is known as cirrhosis. In the early stages, the main symptoms of PBC are due to the accumulation of bile acids and salts in the blood. Patients complain of generalized itching and tiredness. Later on in the disease they develop jaundice (yellow tinge of the skin and the eyes), pale stools, and dark urine. In the late stages, cirrhosis can cause accumulation of fluid in the abdomen (ascites) and internal bleeding from buildup of pressure in the veins of the esophagus (esophageal varices).

The diagnosis is suspected when a patient with Sjogren's has the above symptoms and abnormal liver function tests. There is also a very specific blood test for the diagnosis of PBC, the presence of anti-mitochondrial antibodies. However, a liver biopsy is usually necessary to confirm the diagnosis and to evaluate if the disease is in its early or late stages. This involves taking a small piece of liver, using a needle, under a local anesthetic.

The lack of bile salts in the intestine results in reduced absorption of fat and the fat-soluble vitamins A, D, E, and K. Vitamin D deficiency can result in weakening of the bones (osteoporosis) and fractures. Vitamin K deficiency can result in problems with blood clotting. Therefore patients with PBC benefit from taking calcium plus vitamin D supplements to strengthen their bones, as well as vitamins A, E, and K.

Because the cause of PBC is not known, there is no curative treatment for the disease. The only definite treatment is liver transplantation. However, the prognosis of PBC varies greatly from one patient to another. Many patients lead active lives with few symptoms for 10 to 20 years. In some patients, however, the condition progresses more rapidly and liver failure may occur in just a few years.

Ursodeoxycholic acid may delay the progression of the disease. In large trials, it has been shown to improve liver function as well as survival of patients with PBC. Treatment of pruritis is often a challenge in PBC. The mainstay is cholestyramine, a resin that forms a complex with bile acids in the intestine, promoting their excretion in the stools.

In chronic active hepatitis (CAH), the immune system continuously attacks the liver cells, and as a result, scarring of the liver (cirrhosis) can occur. In general, CAH can be caused by hepatitis viruses, by drugs, or by an unknown mechanism that dysregulates the immune system. The last of these is the case in Sjogren's patients. CAH is suspected in a patient with Sjogren's when liver function tests become abnormal without the patient taking any new drugs. Evidence pointing toward an autoimmune active hepatitis is the finding of antibodies in the blood against smooth muscle or liver/kidney microsomes. Typical symptoms are fatigue, malaise, fever, and loss of appetite. The diagnosis is confirmed by liver biopsy. CAH can be treated by the use of steroids and other immunosuppressive drugs such as azathioprine.

The Heart

Involvement of the heart is very rare in primary Sjogren's. Some Sjogren's patients have been found to have a small amount of fluid around the heart, known as pericardial effusion. This is caused by inflammation of the lining around the heart (pericarditis). It is usually picked up by chance on routine ultrasound scanning of the heart, as most patients are asymptomatic. Patients with secondary Sjogren's who have lupus are more likely to develop pericarditis that gives rise to symptoms. This usually occurs during a lupus flare. The symptoms are typically of left-sided chest pain that changes with posture. When the patient is examined using a stethoscope, a characteristic sound, known as a "rub," can be heard at the left edge of the sternum. An electrocardiogram may show typical changes of pericarditis, and visualization of the heart using echocardiography reveals fluid around the heart. Lupus patients mostly develop small to medium collections of fluid around the heart that have no bearing on the heart function. However, very rarely, if there is a large amount of fluid around the heart, it can impede the pumping action of the heart, and the patient can develop heart failure. Patients with rheumatoid arthritis and secondary Sjogren's can also develop pericardial effusions during a flare of the rheumatoid arthritis. However, it has been estimated that during the course of their disease, less than 10 percent of rheumatoid arthritis patients have a clinical episode of pericarditis.

Steroids are given to treat small to medium pericardial effusions, whereas in the case of large effusions, draining of the fluid using a needle may be necessary.

Congenital Heart Block

When the fetus is inside the womb, its heart beats regularly as a result of its natural pacemaker. However, there is a condition whereby this pacemaker fails and the heart rate drops dangerously low. This is known as congenital heart block. There are two types of congenital heart block, incomplete and complete. In complete heart block, insertion of an artificial pacemaker is necessary after delivery.

All babies born with congenital heart block have mothers who carry anti-Ro/SSA antibodies, whereas 75 percent have mothers with anti-La/SSB antibodies. Most of these mothers have these antibodies without having any symptoms of an autoimmune disease. These antibodies are thought to cross the placenta and bind onto the fetal heart, preventing the normal development of the pacemaker.

Up to 75 percent of Sjogren's patients have anti-Ro/SSA antibodies and up to 40 percent have anti-La/SSB antibodies. However, if a woman who has Sjogren's and anti-Ro/SSA antibodies becomes pregnant, the risk of having a fetus with congenital heart block is only 1–2 percent. The risk is much higher if she has previously given birth to another baby with congenital heart block. For this reason, the fetuses of anti-Ro/SSA- and anti-La/SSB-positive mothers need to be closely monitored after the 18th week of gestation for signs of heart block (see also pages 196–198). If heart block is detected and is of the reversible form, treatment can be given with steroids that cross the placenta (dexamethasone).

The Nervous System

Patients with Sjogren's syndrome can have disease of the nervous system. The peripheral nerves that control sensation can be damaged by the immune system. This is known as sensory neuropathy. Patients with sensory neuropathy initially complain of numbness or tingling at the tips of their toes. Also, they may notice alterations in the appreciation of pain and temperature, and a burning sensation. The problem is usually symmetrical. It can progress very slowly to involve the fingers of both hands. In most patients the symptoms are mild and non-disabling. Approximately 40 percent of patients improve spontaneously.

The diagnosis is usually made by examination of the peripheral nerves. Patients may have reduced sensation in the hands and feet in a "glove and stocking" pattern. The reflexes may also be absent. However, the physical examination can be normal. The diagnosis is confirmed by electrical stimulation tests, called nerve conduction studies. As most patients have mild symptoms, no specific treatment is usually given for peripheral sensory neuropathy in Sjogren's. For patients with severe symptoms, treatment may prove difficult. There are some therapies that can be tried, such as intravenous immunoglobulin or plasmapheresis.

Sometimes an individual nerve that controls the movement of one muscle can be affected, and this can result in weakness of the muscle. One such example is if a patient suddenly develops foot drop on one side. This is known as mononeuritis. The cause of this problem is inflammation in the blood vessel supplying the individual nerve or vasculitis. Vasculitis can be treated by the use of steroids or other drugs that suppress the immune system. If the treatment is given early, the nerve can recover from the damage and the muscle weakness can resolve.

The cranial nerves, that is, the nerves supplying the face, can also be affected in Sjogren's. Most commonly the sensory branch of the trigeminal nerve is affected. This supplies the sensation around the eyes, the nose, the cheeks, and the mouth. In Sjogren's, the symptoms of trigeminal neuropathy are numbness or tingling around the mouth and the cheeks. The area around the eye is less commonly involved. Pain may be present but usually is not severe.

In carpal tunnel syndrome, a common complication in Sjogren's, inflamed tissue in the forearm presses against the median nerve, causing pain, numbness, tingling, and sometimes muscle weakness in the thumb and index and middle fingers. The symptoms are often worse at night. The diagnosis is confirmed by nerve conduction studies. Night splints can help alleviate the symptoms. Also, steroid injections into the carpal tunnel can give temporary relief for up to few months. Steroid injections can be repeated once or twice, but if the symptoms persist, surgery may be necessary. The surgical procedure, known as carpal tunnel decompression, involves making a small cut on the inside of the wrist to free the tissues that press the median nerve. This can be done under local anesthetic on an outpatient basis. It is usually very successful.

Sjogren's has been reported to affect the brain. However, this point will remain controversial until further studies are done. In studies of Sjogren's patients all over the world, a variety of neurological symptoms originating from the brain have been recorded. For example, some patients have been noted to have symptoms of epilepsy, stroke, multiple sclerosis, or Parkinson's disease. However, there is no consensus as to the proportion of Sjogren's patients affected by diseases of the brain. Although these neurological diseases are noted to occur in Sjogren's patients, they may not necessarily be caused by Sjogren's.

Some Sjogren's patients have been noted to have memory or concentration problems or symptoms of anxiety and depression. Again, the percentages quoted in studies vary (7 to 80 percent). Part of the problem is that the symptoms can be quite subtle and not easily recognized. Memory or concentration problems can also sometimes be a manifestation of anxiety or depression, so patients have to be carefully evaluated by a psychologist or psychiatrist. If anxiety or depression is confirmed, therapy in the form of psychological counseling or drugs (antidepressants) may be of benefit. Also, patients with isolated memory or concentration problems may improve with the help of mental exercises prescribed by specially trained psychologists.

TABLE 10.1 ORGAN INVOLVEMENT IN PATIENTS WITH PRIMARY SJOGREN'S

Organ	Complication	Percentage of patients with primary Sjogren's also affected by this complication
Lung	Interstitial lung disease	6 percent
Lung	Small-airway disease	23 percent
Lung	Pleurisy	2 percent
Kidney	Interstitial nephritis	9 percent
Esophagus	Esophageal dysmotility	36 percent
Heart	Pericarditis	2 percent
Liver	Primary biliary cirrhosis	4 percent
Nerves	Carpal tunnel syndrome	12 percent
Nerves	Peripheral neuropathy	2 percent

Summing Up

The major body organs can be affected in one-third of primary Sjogren's patients. Involvement of the lungs usually produces mild symptoms not requiring other than symptomatic treatment. Interstitial lung disease occurs rarely and requires treatment with steroids and immunosuppressive drugs. Involvement of the kidneys can manifest itself as interstitial nephritis which is usually benign and requires no treatment. Very rarely it may cause kidney damage, which can be reversed if treated early with steroids. More severe disease such as glomerulonephritis can sometimes occur, requiring treatment with steroids and immunosuppressive drugs. Esophageal dysmotility can cause difficulty in swallowing as well as acid reflux. The latter can be treated with drugs that reduce acid production by the stomach. More rarely, indigestion can be due to atrophic gastritis. This can result in pernicious anemia that can be treated with regular vitamin B_{12} injections.

Primary biliary cirrhosis can rarely occur in association with Sjogren's and has a variable prognosis. Ursodeoxycholic acid can delay the progression of the disease. Chronic active hepatitis can also rarely occur, and it can be treated with steroids and immunosuppressive drugs. Pericarditis usually occurs in patients with secondary Sjogren's and systemic lupus erythematosus and can be successfully treated with steroids. The most common disease of the peripheral nerves in Sjogren's is carpal tunnel syndrome. It can be treated with steroid injections or surgery. Peripheral sensory neuropathy can occur in Sjogren's and is usually mild and non-disabling. Very rarely vasculitis can result in mononeuritis, and this can be reversed after treatment with steroids and immunosuppressive drugs. Involvement of the brain is controversial. A variety of symptoms such as memory problems, anxiety, and depression are more common in Sjogren's patients. Other more severe symptoms of epilepsy, stroke, and multiple sclerosis have been reported and may possibly be caused by Sjogren's (see Table 10.1).

Frederick B. Vivino, MD, MS, FACR

11 Manifestations of Connective Tissue Diseases Seen in Secondary Sjogren's

MANY PATIENTS WITH A VARIETY of autoimmune conditions demonstrate manifestations of Sjogren's syndrome. This chapter briefly reviews these and shows how Sjogren's relates with and interacts with them.

Definitions and Terms

The term *connective tissue disorders*, also known as *collagen vascular diseases*, refers to a group of chronic, autoimmune, rheumatic, and systemic inflammatory diseases characterized by the production of auto-antibodies in the blood and inflammation of the connective tissues (what holds us together). Common symptoms include arthritis, musculoskeletal pain, Raynaud's phenomenon (see below), skin rashes, fatigue, interstitial lung disease (scarring of the lungs), esophageal dysmotility (disordered contraction of the esophagus), and reflux. Other internal organs may also be affected. The most important connective tissue disorders besides Sjogren's include rheumatoid arthritis, systemic lupus erythematosus, scleroderma, polymyositis, dermatomyositis, mixed connective tissue disease, undifferentiated connective tissue disease, and vasculitis, and will be briefly discussed in this chapter.

When a previously healthy person develops dry eye and dry mouth associated with autoantibodies in the blood or a positive lip biopsy, he or she will be diagnosed with primary Sjogren's syndrome. When a person has a known connective tissue disease (e.g., rheumatoid arthritis for five years) and then later develops dry eye and dry mouth as a further complication, we call it secondary Sjogren's syndrome (i.e., secondary to another connective tissue disease). The ratio of patients with primary and secondary Sjogren's is roughly 1:1. Other autoimmune disorders that primarily affect a single organ system may coexist with primary Sjogren's syndrome but are not strictly classed among the connective tissue diseases. These include Hashimoto's thyroiditis, Raynaud's, and antiphospholipid antibody syndrome.

Rheumatoid Arthritis

Rheumatoid arthritis (RA) is the most common autoimmune rheumatic disease and may affect up to 1–1.5 percent of the North American population. It occurs most often in people 40–60 years old but may develop at any age, even in children. The female-to-male ratio is 2.5 to 1. As the name implies, the target organ for inflammation in RA is the joint, particularly the joint lining or synovium. Rheumatoid arthritis patients typically develop painful swelling of small and large joints over a period of weeks to months. A symmetrical polyarthritis develops over time. In rare cases this process occurs more acutely. The proximal interphalangeal (PIP) and metacarpalphalangeal (MCP) joints (the knuckles closest to the wrist) of the hands, the wrists, elbows, shoulders, hips, knees, ankles, and feet are usually affected. The arthritis is associated with fatigue and generalized morning stiffness. The daily stiffness often limits patient mobility and lasts 45–60 minutes or longer before maximal improvement. In some cases, subcutaneous nodules (rheumatoid nodules) develop around the elbows or at pressure points in the extremities.

The diagnosis of RA is based on clinical findings and results of laboratory studies, X-rays, and joint fluid analysis. The latter test is performed by aspirating synovial fluid from a swollen joint to look for inflammation (i.e., WBC count > 2,000/mm^3) and to exclude infectious causes of arthritis and the presence of crystals as seen in polyarticular gout and pseudorheumatoid pseudogout, two disorders that can mimic RA. Diagnosis of RA requires the presence of symptoms and signs for at least six weeks (Table 11.1). Serum rheumatoid factor is positive in 70–80 percent of patients at onset and 90 percent of patients in advanced cases. Although helpful in diagnosis, serum rheumatoid factor is

---

TABLE 11.1   CRITERIA FOR THE CLASSIFICATION OF RHEUMATOID ARTHRITIS

---

1. Morning stiffness ≥ 1 hour
2. Arthritis of ≥ 3 joint areas
3. Arthritis of hand joints (PIPs, MCPs) or wrists
4. Symmetric arthritis
5. Rheumatoid nodules
6. Serum rheumatoid factor
7. Radiographic changes (erosions, periarticular demineralization)

Note: Criteria 1–4 must be present for at least 6 weeks. Classification or diagnosis as RA requires 4 of 7 criteria.
Source: Modified from *Arthritis Rheum* 1988; 31;315–324.

not specific for the disease and may occur in primary Sjogren's syndrome and other connective tissue diseases. X-rays show symmetric narrowing of joint spaces due to cartilage loss, thinning of bone around inflamed joints (periarticular demineralization), and erosions. Erosions (little holes at the edges of the bone ends) develop as early as one year after onset and exemplify the destructive nature of RA. Patients with primary Sjogren's can also develop a rheumatoid-like arthritis, but erosions are not typically observed.

In a subset of patients the inflammation spreads to other organs and causes secondary Sjogren's syndrome and other problems. The most common morbidities include scleritis and episcleritis (inflammation of the outer layers of the ocular surface), interstitial lung disease, pleural and pericardial effusions (fluid around the lungs or heart), cutaneous vasculitis (inflammation of blood vessels), carpal tunnel syndrome, peripheral neuropathy, and cervical subluxation with myelopathy (spinal cord injury due to unstable neck bones).

Most cases of rheumatoid arthritis require aggressive treatment, including multiple medications and physical therapy, to prevent disability, deformity, and other complications. Non-steroidal anti-inflammatory drugs (NSAIDs) (e.g., ibuprofen), oral and intraarticular steroids, hydroxychloroquine, methotrexate, and the TNF-α inhibitors (etanercept, infliximab, adalimumab) are the most commonly used treatments. Patients who fail medical therapy eventually may require joint replacement surgery.

TABLE 11.2   CRITERIA FOR THE CLASSIFICATION OF SYSTEMIC LUPUS ERYTHEMATOSUS

---

1. Malar rash
2. Discoid rash
3. Photosensitivity
4. Oral ulcers
5. Arthritis
6. Serositis
7. Renal disorder
8. Neurologic disorder
9. Hematologic disorder
10. Abnormal immunology test
11. Antinuclear antibody positivity

Note: Classification as SLE requires that 4 of 11 criteria be met.
Source: Modified from *Arthritis Rheum* 1982, 25;1271-7.

Systemic Lupus Erythematosus

Systemic lupus erythematosus (SLE) is a chronic autoimmune rheumatic disorder characterized by immune complex (antigen-antibody complex) deposition in various tissues, causing multiple organ disease and/or failure in association with anti-nuclear antibody (ANA) production in the blood. In North America lupus affects approximately 0.05 percent of the general population and preferentially strikes young women (the female-to-male ratio is 8:1) in the 15–40 age group, especially African Americans. Less commonly SLE occurs among men, pediatric patients, and older adults. Lupus often runs in families.

Because lupus patients may manifest a myriad of medical problems, diagnosis can be challenging. However, the American College of Rheumatology has advanced a set of research classification criteria that also provide a useful framework for diagnosis (Table 11.2). The criteria recognize the high prevalence of mucocutaneous manifestations and auto-antibody production in the disease. Four of eleven criteria must be satisfied either simultaneously or sequentially for classification as SLE. Since some patients don't exhibit the full-blown syndrome at disease onset, the diagnosis of lupus is sometimes suspected but not unequivocally confirmed until months or years later.

Lupus causes a variety of skin rashes, including hives, blisters, a measles-like rash, and a rash that resembles psoriasis. The most characteristic skin and mucous membrane abnormalities, however, include the malar rash, discoid rash, skin photosensitivity, oral ulcers, or nasal ulcers. The malar or butterfly rash looks like a red patch over the nasal bridge, nose, and cheeks in the shape of a butterfly and heals without scarring. In contrast, discoid lupus causes raised, red plaques on the head and extremities. These plaques are often associated with scaling and follicular plugging, and heal with loss of pigmentation, scarring, and/or loss of hair. In some instances patients with lupus develop severe skin rashes in sun-exposed areas (photosensitive rashes) following brief exposure to the sun or ultraviolet light. Painless or painful oral and nasal ulcers can also occur, especially in individuals with active skin disease.

The diagnostic hallmark of SLE is the presence of antinuclear antibodies (ANAs), found in up to 95 percent of patients when tested by indirect immunofluorescence using the Hep-2 cell substrate. Cases of ANA-negative lupus (i.e., patients with clinical lupus but a negative test) can be diagnosed by testing for anti-Ro/SSA and anti-La/SSB using a different assay system. This is because the marker autoantibodies for Sjogren's syndrome, anti-La/SSB and anti-Ro/SSA, are also found in 15–45 percent of SLE patients. Anti-Sm antibodies are most specific for SLE but are found in < 30 percent of patients. Anti-double-stranded-DNA antibodies occur in < 60 percent of patients and correlate best with disease activity, especially lupus kidney disease. Titers tend to rise with disease flares and fall toward normal with improvement. In contrast, levels of complement (immune mediator proteins) C3, C4, and CH50 tend to fall with disease exacerbations (as immune complexes are formed and bind complement) but rise with remissions. Lupus patients also form antibodies to phospholipids, and this will sometimes cause a false positive RPR or VDRL blood test for syphilis. The ANA and other immunologic tests are two of the necessary four criteria for diagnosis.

Constitutional symptoms in lupus include fevers, weight loss, malaise, and fatigue. Internal organ involvement in SLE also causes serious and sometimes life-threatening complications. Interstitial lung disease, pleurisy (inflammation of the lining around the lung), pleural effusions, inflammatory pneumonitis (pneumonia), and pulmonary hemorrhage all cause shortness of breath and, in the most severe cases, lead to respiratory failure. Pericarditis (inflammation of the heart lining) and pericardial effusions cause chest pain and shortness of breath. Heart failure, valvular heart disease, and accelerated coronary atherosclerosis also occur. Acute or chronic kidney inflammation (lupus nephritis) due to glomerulonephritis (inflammation of the kidney filtration units) or inter-stitial nephritis (inflammation of the tissues surrounding the glomeruli) leads to loss of kidney function and the appearance of protein, cells, and/or casts in the urine. In the most severe cases lupus nephritis may rapidly progress and necessitate prompt diagnosis and treatment to pre-vent the need for dialysis or even patient demise.

Critical complications can also develop with central nervous system involvement. Lupus can cause seizures, psychosis, coma, stroke, mini-stroke, mood disorders, confusion, cognitive dysfunction, chorea (move-ment disorders), transverse myelitis (spinal cord damage due to inflam-mation), and abnormalities of the cranial nerves. Peripheral neuropathies also occur. The musculoskeletal manifestations of lupus include arthral-gias and myalgias (joint and muscle pain) along with polyarthritis. The arthritis of SLE can cause deformities similar to those seen in rheumatoid arthritis but rarely causes erosions. Hematologic abnormalities in lupus include autoimmune hemolytic anemia and thrombocytopenia (low platelets). In these conditions the body forms antibodies against its own red blood cells or platelets, and patients develop fatigue, shortness of breath, or bleeding.

The ten-year survival rate in lupus is approximately 90 percent, and many patients have mild cases (e.g., skin rashes, joint pain) that do not require treatment with toxic drugs. Skin rashes, hair loss, and oral ulcers can be effectively managed with hydroxychloroquine, other anti-malarial drugs, and/or topical steroids. Hydroxychloroquine and NSAIDs alle-viate arthritis and joint and muscle pain. Use of oral steroids (e.g., pred-nisone), intravenous steroids, and/or more toxic immunosuppressives (e.g., azathioprine, cyclophosphamide) is indicated in patients who fail more conservative measures or develop life-threatening problems such as hemolytic anemia, severe thrombocytopenia, or disease of the heart, lungs, kidneys, or central nervous system.

Antiphospholipid Antibody Syndrome

Antiphospholipid antibody syndrome (APS) is an autoimmune dis-order characterized by recurrent arterial and venous thromboses (blood clots) and/or recurrent spontaneous abortions (miscarriages) associated with the presence of antibodies to phospholipids. It can occur by itself as a primary disorder (primary APS) or in association with connective tissue disease (secondary APS), most notably lupus. Its occurrence in primary Sjogren's syndrome is infrequent. It most commonly causes deep venous thromboses in the arms and legs, pulmonary emboli (clots in the lungs), strokes, mini-strokes or recurrent miscarriages (usually in the second or third trimester). Blood clots must be documented by objective medical testing, and antibody presence is demonstrated when one or more of the following blood tests is positive: anticardiolipin antibodies, lupus anticoagulant, or anti-beta-2-glycoprotein I. Mild thrombocytopenia also occurs in APS but doesn't prevent clots. The major treatment is lifelong anticoagulation with blood thinners such as heparin or warfarin. Other causes of blood clots and pregnancy loss must always be excluded in the diagnostic evaluation. The antibodies may occasionally occur in normal people and don't always cause clots when present.

Scleroderma

As the name implies, scleroderma, or systemic sclerosis, is a multisystem autoimmune rheumatic disease characterized by progressive thickening and induration of the skin in association with fibrosis (scarring) of the internal organs and thickening of small blood vessels. It affects a small percentage of the general population (0.02–0.075 percent), with peak occurrence at ages 35–65 years and a female preponderance. In early stages it causes puffiness of the hands, later followed by skin thickening on the fingers and toes. The skin on the digits becomes tight and shiny like leather (sclerodactyly), and this process gradually spreads up the arms and legs to involve the face and occasionally the trunk as well. Diagnosis can be made by skin biopsy or documentation of skin involvement and typical features by an experienced clinician. Diagnosis of scleroderma requires the presence of one major and two minor criteria (Table 11.3).

Patients are classified into disease subsets and prognostic categories according to the degree of clinically involved skin and autoantibody profile. People with limited scleroderma have cutaneous thickening of the distal limbs (below the elbows and knees) without truncal involvement and are typically anti-centromere antibody positive (40–50 percent). The CREST syndrome (calcinosis, Raynaud's, esophageal dysmotility, sclerodactyly, telangiectasias) falls within the classification scheme of limited systemic sclerosis. People with diffuse scleroderma have skin thickening

---

TABLE 11.3   CRITERIA FOR THE CLASSIFICATION OF SYSTEMIC SCLEROSIS

A. Major: Symmetric thickening, tightening and induration of skin above the metacarpal-phalangeal joints (where the fingers join the hands) or metatarsal-phalangeal joints (where the toes join the feet)
B. Minor:
    1. Sclerodactyly
    2. Scarring of finger tips or loss of finger pads
    3. Chest X-ray scarring at the base of both lungs

Note: Classification of scleroderma requires one major or two minor criteria.
Source: Modified from *Arthritis Rheum*, 1980, 23;581–590.

above and below the elbows, knees, and/or trunk. They are typically anti-scleroderma or anti-Scl-70 antibody positive (20–30 percent) and carry a worse prognosis due to greater internal organ disease. Raynaud's phenomenon (cold-induced color changes in the fingers) is discussed further below and may predate the onset of scleroderma by months to years.

When the skin thickening begins, patients can also develop itching, malaise, fatigue, arthritis, and musculoskeletal pain. Scarring of the gastrointestinal tract causes difficulty swallowing due to esophageal dysmotility (disordered contractions of the esophagus) and severe gastroesophageal reflux disease (GERD). Interstitial fibrosis and pulmonary hypertension (high blood pressure in the lungs) lead to progressive shortness of breath, especially during exertion. Pericarditis, pericardial effusions, heart rhythm abnormalities, and heart failure result from inflammation and scarring of cardiac tissue. Hypertension associated with acute renal failure, also called scleroderma renal crisis, is a medical emergency that may necessitate dialysis or cause patient demise. Muscle weakness due to myositis (muscle inflammation) can also occur.

Symptomatic treatments are available and used according to organ involvement. Some patients will note spontaneous improvement of skin thickening over time or following use of medications such as D-penicillamine or methotrexate. Reflux is treated by diet and use of proton pump inhibitors (e.g., omeprazole). Angiotensin-converting enzyme (ACE) inhibitors (e.g., captopril) can control blood pressure and preserve kidney function if initiated early in scleroderma renal crisis.

Raynaud's Phenomenon

Raynaud's phenomenon is defined as cold-induced color changes of the fingers, toes, nose, or earlobes that result from spasm and/or thickening of small arteries at involved sites. It can exist as an isolated problem (primary Raynaud's disease) or in association with any of the connective tissue disorders including Sjogren's (secondary Raynaud's). It causes the worst problems among individuals with scleroderma. Patients typically develop blanching of part of the fingers or involved areas after exposure to cold, followed by cyanosis (bluing) and later erythema (redness) upon rewarming. Occasionally, episodes can be induced by nicotine from cigarette smoke or emotional stress. Primary Raynaud's disease usually affects young women and may be annoying to the patient but seldom causes significant discomfort or permanent damage. In contrast, secondary Raynaud's may cause ischemic pain and/or numbness followed eventually by complications such as digital ulcers, infections, loss of the fingertip pads or bone, and digital gangrene. Patients are treated with calcium channel blockers (e.g., nifedipine) to relax the blood vessels and with anti-platelet agents (e.g., aspirin) to prevent clots. The most severe cases will require use of intravenous medications, nerve blocks, or surgical amputation.

Polymyositis and Dermatomyositis

Polymyositis and dermatomyositis comprise a group of autoimmune rheumatic diseases that cause skeletal muscle weakness and inflammation (myositis). Dermatomyositis also causes a characteristic rash. These disorders affect 0.05–0.08 percent of the population with peak age at onset of 10–15 years in children and 45–60 years in adults. The female-to-male ratio is 2:1. Polymyositis is more common than dermatomyositis in adults, and the reverse is true for children.

Patients insidiously develop symmetric weakness of proximal muscles around the shoulders and hips over a three- to- six-month period. This may cause difficulty getting up from a chair, climbing stairs, walking, or raising an arm to comb the hair or hang up a coat. The myositis may spread to muscles that control breathing or swallowing and cause shortness of breath or dysphagia (difficulty swallowing). Other problems include fatigue, arthritis, joint and muscle pain, Raynaud's, interstitial lung disease, GERD, esophageal dysmotility, and heart failure. Secondary

Sjogren's can also complicate polymyositis and dermatomyositis, and myositis can occasionally be a manifestation of primary Sjogren's.

People with dermatomyositis exhibit one or more of several characteristics rashes. These include the heliotrope rash (lilac discoloration of the eyelids), Gottron's sign (a scaly, red rash over the knuckles), shawl sign (redness of the posterior shoulders and neck), and the V-sign (redness of the anterior neck and upper chest). Children with dermatomyositis often develop ectopic calcifications (painful calcium deposits of the skeletal muscle and subcutaneous tissues). The diagnosis of polymyositis or dermatomyositis is suspected when the skeletal muscle enzymes, creatine phosphokinase (CPK) and aldolase, are elevated in the blood of a patient who is weak. An electromyographic or EMG study will demonstrate abnormal electrical activity of the muscles and help eliminate a neuropathy as the cause of the weakness. The diagnosis is confirmed by biopsy of an involved muscle that shows damage and infiltration of muscle fibers by lymphocytes and other inflammatory cells.

Although not found in the majority of patients, the presence of certain myositis-specific autoantibodies suggests disease correlates. Anti-Jo 1 antibodies denote a subset of polymyositis patients with the anti-synthetase syndrome (fever, Raynaud's, interstitial lung disease, polyarthritis), while anti-SRP (signal recognition particle) antibodies in polymyositis suggest a poor prognosis and response to treatment. Anti-PM-1 (or anti-PM-Scl) antibodies are found in patients with a scleroderma-myositis overlap syndrome, while anti-Mi-2 antibodies are observed in patients with classic dermatomyositis.

Most patients with polymyositis or dermatomyositis respond to treatment with high-dose oral and/or intravenous steroids followed by physical therapy for gait training and muscle strengthening. Patients who fail steroids or develop unacceptable side effects may be treated with other immunosuppressive agents, including methotrexate, azathioprine, cyclosporine, and intravenous gamma globulin.

Mixed Connective Tissue Disease

Mixed connective tissue disease, as originally described, denotes a subset of connective tissue disease patients whose blood contains high titers of anti-RNP (ribonucleoprotein) antibodies. Antinuclear antibodies and rheumatoid factor are also observed. Patients typically manifest features of several different connective tissue diseases, including RA, SLE, scleroderma, and polymyositis or dermatomyositis. Secondary Sjogren's may also occur. The most common signs and symptoms include puffy hands, sclerodactyly, Raynaud's, skin rashes, pleurisy, polyarthritis, dysphagia, reflux, myalgias, and myositis. Most patients evolve into classic lupus or scleroderma over time, and autoantibody profiles may change. When patients meet diagnostic criteria for two different collagen vascular diseases at the time of diagnosis, the term *overlap syndrome* is preferred.

Undifferentiated Connective Tissue Disease

This term describes a group of individuals who exhibit signs and symptoms of connective tissue disease and are ANA positive but anti-RNP negative. These patients fail to meet the diagnostic criteria for any one specific disorder. They may complain of sicca symptoms, but lip biopsies are typically negative. In some cases, a change over time in clinical features or autoantibody profile may yield a specific diagnosis.

Vasculitis

Vasculitis is a broad term that describes a heterogeneous group of collagen vascular disorders that cause blood vessel inflammation with subsequent damage to the vessel wall, tissue necrosis from ischemia (poor blood supply), and in some cases eventual organ failure. Its clinical manifestations vary according to the site of involvement. It can be localized to a single organ or cause systemic disease. Vasculitis can exist as a primary disorder (e.g., polyarteritis nodosa) or occur as a complication of another connective tissue disease, including Sjogren's syndrome. It can sometimes be precipitated by infections or medication side effects. Vasculitic disorders are grouped according to (1) the size and type of vessel involved, (2) the type of cells that cause the vessel inflammation, (3) etiology, and (4) affected organs.

The subset of Sjogren's syndrome patients with extraglandular manifestations (i.e., serious internal organ disease; see Chapter 10) are also the individuals at greatest risk for the development of vasculitis. Laboratory clues may include the appearance of cryoglobulins in the blood (proteins that precipitate out in the cold); high titers of anti-Ro/SSA antibodies; elevation of serum IgG, gamma globulins, or the erythrocyte sedimentation rate; low levels of complement C3 or C4; or positive antineutrophil cytoplasmic (ANCA) antibodies. However, as with other patient groups, the definitive diagnosis of vasculitis in Sjogren's can only be made by biopsy of an involved organ or by doing an arteriogram. The biopsy should show invasion and/or damage of blood vessel walls by inflammatory cells. The arteriogram is performed by injecting radio-opaque contrast dye into an artery to look for abnormalities of vessel shape, including aneurysms, segmental narrowing, or dilatation.

The skin is the most frequent site of vasculitis in Sjogren's syndrome. Cutaneous vasculitis affects small vessels (arterioles, capillaries, venules) and typically causes raised reddish purple spots on the legs, called palpable purpura. These lesions may be painful or pruritic. Other vasculitic rashes in Sjogren's include urticaria (hives), skin ulcers, or erythema multiforme (red spots of variable size and shape). Vasculitic involvement of small to medium arteries in Sjogren's syndrome will occasionally affect the nervous system and cause strokes, mini-strokes, or peripheral neuropathies. A particular type of peripheral neuropathy, mononeuritis multiplex, is highly suggestive of vasculitis and is suspected when the patient develops foot drop associated with patchy loss of sensation in the lower extremities. The diagnosis is confirmed by performing an EMG/nerve conduction study of the legs followed by biopsy of the sural nerve. Vasculitis of the medium-sized arteries of abdominal organs is rare in Sjogren's syndrome but can cause life-threatening complications. The diagnosis is proven by arteriogram or examination of tissue specimens obtained during emergency surgery.

Treatments for vasculitis vary with the organs involved but in some cases prove to be long, difficult, and extremely toxic. Therefore, every effort should be made to obtain a proper diagnosis at the time of initial presentation and exclude other disorders that cause similar symptoms but require different treatments.

Secondary Sjogren's Syndrome: Clinical Manifestations, Diagnosis, and Prevalence

The onset of secondary Sjogren's syndrome among connective tissue disease patients is highly variable (1–40 years) but occurs in the majority of people about 5–10 years after diagnosis of the primary, underlying disorder. Sicca symptoms in secondary Sjogren's are generally milder than those of primary Sjogren's. It remains unclear whether this phenomenon reflects lesser severity or earlier diagnosis facilitated as a benefit of rheumatologic care for other problems. Clearly, however, the prevalence of salivary gland swelling, adenopathy (swelling of the lymph nodes), and lymphomas in secondary Sjogren's is diminished compared to its primary counterpart.

Some studies suggest that dry eye occurs more commonly than dry mouth in lupus and RA patients with secondary Sjogren's, while in scleroderma patients with secondary Sjogren's, the reverse seems true. Interestingly, in scleroderma, secondary Sjogren's occurs more commonly among the limited variant than the diffuse form of the disease. Treatments for these patient groups are typically directed toward the underlying disease. However, symptomatic patients with secondary Sjogren's may also benefit from therapy with secretogogues and other measures, as discussed in Chapters 14 and 15.

At the present time, the diagnosis of secondary Sjogren's is most easily accomplished by utilizing the revised European-American classification criteria that were recently adopted by the Sjogren's Syndrome Foundation (see Table 2.2). These require that patients have an established connective tissue disease, at least one sicca symptom, and two out of three objective tests for dry eye and dry mouth.

The prevalence of secondary Sjogren's in other collagen vascular disorders remains controversial and depends on how this diagnosis is made. When older diagnostic criteria were applied to large patient populations, prevalence figures for secondary Sjogren's of 31 percent, 20 percent, and 20 percent were reported in patients with rheumatoid arthritis, lupus, and scleroderma, respectively. According to one survey, anti-Ro/SSA and anti-La/SSB are normally present in primary Sjogren's and lupus, as described above, but become more prevalent in all patient groups with the development of secondary Sjogren's: rheumatoid arthritis (24 percent/6 percent), lupus (73 percent/46 percent), and scleroderma (33 percent/18 percent). Studies of positive lip biopsies in the same patient groups suggest prevalence figures that are even higher: RA 35 percent, SLE 18–90 percent, and scleroderma 17–51 percent. Interestingly, the proportion of patients with positive biopsies in these studies was always substantially higher than the number of patients with symptoms. Perhaps future studies of prevalence utilizing the new classification criteria will settle this controversy.

How Sjogren's Syndrome May Influence the Expression of Other Connective Tissue Diseases

The influence of secondary Sjogren's on the course of other connective tissue diseases has not been closely examined. In rheumatoid arthritis patients the coexistence of secondary Sjogren's reportedly has little effect on the course of arthritis or other clinical manifestations. However, dryness of the gastrointestinal tract from Sjogren's syndrome could potentially exacerbate a variety of problems common to these disorders, including reflux, dysphagia, dyspepsia (upset stomach), and constipation. Respiratory dryness from Sjogren's could not only aggravate chronic cough due to interstitial lung disease but also predispose to recurrent respiratory infections. In lupus, two studies suggest that secondary Sjogren's is associated with an increased incidence of erosive polyarthritis, an uncommon complication of SLE. In scleroderma, a study of over 800 people reported that patients with systemic sclerosis and secondary Sjogren's (particularly the CREST variant) were at increased risk of developing vasculitis. Another study reported that autoimmune liver disease, particularly primary biliary cirrhosis, was more prevalent in scleroderma patients with secondary Sjogren's compared to scleroderma patients alone. Further studies will shed additional light on these observations.

Evolution of Sjogren's Syndrome into Other Disorders

As alluded to previously, patients with various connective tissue disorders, including Sjogren's syndrome, share overlapping clinical and laboratory features and are sometimes difficult to tell apart. Rheumatoid arthritis, for example, may be complicated by secondary Sjogren's, and the initial manifestations of primary Sjogren's can include a rheumatoid-like polyarthritis with rheumatoid factor in the blood. Sjogren's syndrome was once thought to be a benign variant of lupus, and the presence of anti-Ro/SSA and anti-La/SSB antibodies in both diseases suggests a common pathogenetic mechanism. Reports also exist in the medical literature of patients who met criteria for both diseases at the time of presentation and were therefore felt to have an SLE-Sjogren's overlap syndrome. Not surprisingly, there are even reports of individuals who started with one disease and evolved into another.

One study from France described 55 patients who presented with sicca symptoms, anti-Ro/SSA or anti-La/SSB, and other manifestations of connective tissue disease and who fulfilled the European diagnostic criteria for primary Sjogren's. Other autoantibodies tested negative. During a subsequent period of 12–14 years, four patients developed new signs and symptoms (malar rash, pleuropericarditis, glomerulonephritis) thought to be atypical for Sjogren's. Follow-up testing revealed the presence of anti-Sm (two patients) and anti-double-stranded DNA (two patients) antibodies, and these patients were eventually diagnosed with lupus according to the American College of Rheumatology criteria. In another report a patient with primary Sjogren's syndrome (dry eye, dry mouth, anti-Ro/SSA, anti-La/SSB) turned anti-centromere positive about three years after he developed parotid swelling and renal tubular acidosis (failure of the kidneys to excrete acid form the blood). He was eventually diagnosed with the CREST variant of scleroderma following the onset of Raynaud's phenomenon, digital ischemia, nail fold capillary dropout, and telangiectasias (dilated small vessels in the skin that cause red spots). Thus, in clinical situations where new symptoms cannot be explained by a previous diagnosis, further evaluation and consideration of a new diagnosis may be necessary.

Other Autoimmune Disorders Associated with Sjogren's Syndrome

Any patient with known autoimmune disease is at increased risk for developing a second autoimmune disorder. This must also be considered when new health problems occur. Other autoimmune disorders found in Sjogren's syndrome patients include celiac sprue, primary biliary cirrhosis, chronic active autoimmune hepatitis, myasthenia gravis, pernicious anemia, multiple sclerosis, Addison's disease, Graves' disease, and Hashimoto's thyroiditis. Hashimoto's thyroiditis most commonly coexists with Sjogren's syndrome and causes goiter and hypothyroidism. It can be difficult to diagnose because symptoms begin insidiously and overlap with those of primary Sjogren's. These may include fatigue, dry skin, coarse hair, constipation, headaches, arthralgias, myalgias, facial swelling, cognitive dysfunction, and hoarseness. Hypothyroidism is diagnosed by blood tests (high TSH, low or normal free T4) and may also occur coincidentally in a Sjogren's patient due to other causes. The diagnosis of Hashimoto's is confirmed by the presence of one or more thyroid autoantibodies in the blood, including anti-microsomal and anti-thyroid peroxidase antibodies. It is treated with thyroid hormone replacement, and frequent monitoring of thyroid function tests is required.

Summing Up

Between 20 and 40 percent of patients with rheumatoid arthritis, lupus, and scleroderma and to a lesser extent other autoimmune disorders also have Sjogren's syndrome. Each of these conditions presents unique challenges that impact the diagnosis and management of the syndrome.

Roger A. Levy

Veronica S. Vilela, MD

Mirhelen M. Abreu, MD

12 Useful Studies: Blood Tests, Imaging, Biopsies, and Beyond

THE REVISED EUROPEAN DIAGNOSTIC criteria of primary Sjogren's syndrome includes anti-Ro/SSA and/or anti-La/SSB antibodies as one of the six items. The antinuclear antibody (ANA) test is a commonly performed serologic assay for aiding in the diagnosis of a few systemic autoimmune diseases, such as systemic lupus erythematosus (SLE), scleroderma, mixed connective tissue disease, and Sjogren's. The test is based on an immune fluorescent technique and is in most instances dependent on a subjective analysis. When ANA is positive, it does not mean that an autoimmune disease is present; it can occur in relatives of patients with a definite diagnosis and in healthy individuals (usually in the lower titer range), and it can also be induced by certain drugs (such as the anti-hypertension agent hydralazine or the psychiatric drug chlorpromazine). When anti-Ro/SSA and/or anti-La/SSB antibodies are present in the serum, the ANA displays a speckled pattern in the cell nuclei. In addition to anti-Ro/SSA and/or anti-La/SSB antibodies, several other laboratory tests are used in the diagnostic investigation of Sjogren's. Once the diagnosis is confirmed, laboratory tests are important in the clinical follow-up of Sjogren's patients and help the rheumatologist and other specialists caring for the Sjogren's patient to evaluate if the disease is flaring up; in addition, some have prognostic value. Since there has been rapid progress in the sensitivity and specificity of several tests and the replacement of a few "old favorites," such as LE cell detection and imprint ANA, it is crucial for the modern clinician to be up to date with

TABLE 12.1   BLOOD TESTING IN SJOGREN'S SYNDROME

Group	Test
Acute phase reactants	CRP, alpha-1-acid GP, erythrocyte sedimentation rate.
Hematologic tests	CBC, platelet count.
Non-specific immune tests	Total serum IgG and IgM, cryoglobulins, protein electrophoresis.
Non-specific autoantibodies	Rheumatoid factor, ANA, anti-Ro/SSA, anti-La/SSB.
Specific autoantibodies	Anti-M3, anti-fodrin.

Key to abbreviations: CRP = C-reactive protein, alpha-1 acid GP = alpha-1 acid glycoprotein, CBC = complete blood count, ANA = antinuclear antibodies

the most recent tests and methods that the clinical laboratory has to offer. In order to facilitate explanation of the different laboratory tests, they are subdivided according to the methodology applied and their specificity. In certain cases it may be difficult to differentiate primary Sjogren's from SLE, and a laboratory test profile may be useful (Table 12.1).

Acute Phase Reactants

The measurement of acute phase reactants or proteins reflects a systemic inflammatory reaction. These proteins are elevated in response to the systemic inflammatory stimulus and are initially depicted by an increase in the erythrocyte sedimentation rate, a nonspecific test in which values are increased in all inflammatory conditions. The sedimentation rate is often used as a follow-up tool; it is a cheap and easy-to-perform test that can be done without much sophistication and shows increased values when there are more acute phase reactants circulating in the blood. It is important to recall that the sedimentation rate is higher when the patient has significant anemia; this should not be understood as increased production of acute phase reactants. The most commonly measured acute phase reactants nowadays are C-reactive protein (CRP), alpha-1 acid glycoprotein (alpha-1 acid-GP) and serum amyloid A (SAA); these are the first ones to increase after an inflammatory stimulus and to drop once treatment is started or the stimulus is blocked. Other acute phase reactants that can also be measured to evaluate systemic inflammation are immunoglobulins, haptoglobin, fibrinogen, factor VIII, and complement system proteins. Most laboratories around the world are currently performing specific determination of acute phase reactants by more sensitive techniques, such as nephelometry and turbidimetry. These ultrasensitive methodologies used for measuring CRP, alpha-1 acid GP, and SAA make them a reliable tool not only for the initial diagnostic investigation, but also during follow-up for evaluating systemic flare-ups. The protein electrophoresis technique separates proteins according to their molecular weights, and different clones can be depicted clearly. The fractions to where the bands of protein migrate in the gel are named with Greek letters, and while albumin, due to its larger size, appears in the first portion, called alpha, most of the acute phase reactants and proteins involved in the inflammatory response migrate to the gamma region. When many proteins are found in increased amounts in the gamma region, it is called polyclonal hypergammaglobulinemia; the condition indicates that several autoantibodies are being formed, along with increased amounts of circulating acute phase reactants. A monoclonal band indicates an uncontrolled expansion of a certain cell type.

Cryoglobulins

Cryoglobulins are proteins involved in the immune response that are separated through a precipitation under cold temperatures. These proteins can be further analyzed by electrophoresis and other immunological and biochemical techniques and then classified according to their characteristics. Cryoglobulins are related to infection with the hepatitis C virus, cutaneous vasculitis, and hypocomplementemia. Polyclonal and monoclonal mixed cryoglobulinemia (type II) can be found in up to 60 percent of primary Sjogren's patients. The most commonly found proteins are IgG polyclonal and IgM K monoclonal. During follow-up, a switch to type I (monoclonal) cryoglobulinemia might be indicative of the appearance of lymphoma.

Hematologic Alterations

The hematologic alterations found in primary Sjogren's, although nonspecific, might add useful information during the initial investigation. During follow-up of primary Sjogren's these parameters are important in evaluating disease activity as well as drug toxicity. In a recent study by Ramos-Casals and colleagues, with 360 patients (93 percent women) followed from 1994 to 2000, anemia was detected in 20 percent, leucopenia in 16 percent, thrombocytopenia in 13 percent, eosinophilia in

TABLE 12.2   LABORATORY TESTS HELPFUL FOR THE DIAGNOSTIC DIFFERENTIATION OF PRIMARY SJOGREN'S AND SLE

Test	Frequency in primary Sjogren's (%)	Frequency in SLE (%)
Antinuclear antibodies (ANA)	80	98
Rheumatoid factor	70	20
Anti-dsDNA	—	60
Anti-Sm	—	30
Anti-RNP	30–40	>5
Anti-Ro/SSA	70	30
Anti-La/SSB	60	15
Anti-ribosomal P protein	—	20
Anti-cardiolipin	14	30–40

12 percent, lymphopenia in 9 percent, elevated sedimentation rate in 22 percent, hypergammaglobulinemia ($>$ 25 percent) in 22 percent, hypogammaglobulinemia ($<$ 15 percent) in 15 percent, reduced IgG in 8 percent, antiphospholipid antibodies in 13 percent, and monoclonal IgM gammopathy in 22 percent.

Sometimes the diagnosis of secondary Sjogren's within the context of a disease such as SLE, scleroderma, or rheumatoid arthritis (RA) is easy to make, but this is not always the case in the initial differential diagnosis workup to distinguish between primary Sjogren's and other systemic connective tissue disorders. Some laboratory findings, such as ANA, anti-Ro/SSA, and anti-La/SSB, are common to primary Sjogren's and SLE (Table 12.2) and sometimes scleroderma. But there are other antibodies that are specific to SLE, such as anti-dsDNA and anti-Sm, and those that are typical of scleroderma, such as anti-topoisomerase I (Scl-70) and the nucleolar pattern of ANA. We have to bear in mind the notion that a positive ANA (especially in low titers) is not a disease marker and can be found in 5 to 30 percent of the normal population. Rheumatoid factor can be found both in primary Sjogren's or its secondary form and also in RA without Sjogren's.

Rheumatoid Factor

Rheumatoid factor (RF) is a type of autoantibody that binds to the Fc portion of IgG and are important in the immune response. B-cells that produce exist in the circulating lymphocyte pool in a high frequency (approximately 1–2 percent) in normal individuals and in patients with pathological conditions associated with the sustained levels of circulating RF, such as rheumatoid arthritis (RA), Sjogren's, and mixed cryoglobulinemia, associated with hepatitis C virus infection. RFs are induced by many infectious entities (viruses, bacteria, parasites) as a consequence of a secondary immune response to the pathogen, but usually the response in these conditions is transient. RF might be found persistently in 50–70 percent of primary Sjogren's patients, it can be of any of the three major immunoglobulin classes, IgG, IgA or IgM, and it is related to the presence of cryoglobulins. Even though it is a nonspecific finding in Sjogren's, the presence of RF is predictive of systemic organ involvement. Because RF titers do not correlate with disease activity, unlike the acute phase reactants, RFs are not used to monitor disease activity or treatment response. IgA RF is directly related to the extension of the inflammatory infiltrate. The variation of RF frequency in primary Sjogren's among different series may be due to differences in patient population selection, in the classification criteria applied, and in the method used for RF detection. Like the appearance of a monoclonal band in the protein electrophoresis, the disappearance of previously found circulating RF and presence of elevated beta-2-microglobulin in the serum have a predictive value for the detection of lymphoma.

ANA, Anti-Ro/SSA, and Anti-La/SSB

Antinuclear antibodies are detected by immune-fluorescent technique in more than 70 percent of the cases of primary Sjogren's and hence serve as a screening tool in diagnosis. ANAs are found also in the secondary forms of Sjogren's and in other connective tissue disorders without Sjogren's, so they are not specific or highly sensitive for primary Sjogren's. The ANA result is expressed in serum dilution titer, and the immune fluorescence pattern has to be described. The substrate most commonly used for the reaction is the HEp2 cell line, as it has a large nucleus that facilitates the fluorescence reading and it has been standardized in most parts of the world. A finely speckled pattern is associated with anti-Ro/SSA with or without anti-La/SSB, which should be investigated by a more specific methodology, such as counterimmune electrophoresis, immune precipitation, or hemagglutination. Although these two autoantibodies are part of the classification criteria of primary

Sjogren's, they are not specific. The reactivity against Ro/SSA and La/ SSB can also be found in subacute cutaneous SLE and in mothers and infants with so-called neonatal lupus syndrome. A coarse speckled pattern might be related to anti-RNP with or without anti-Sm antibodies, the presence of which should also be confirmed by specific techniques such as the above. In an entity called mixed connective tissue disease (MCTD), anti-RNP antibodies are the only type of autoantibodies found, and the clinical picture is composed of signs and symptoms of SLE, scleroderma, RA, and dermatopolymyositis. When a rim pattern is found around the nucleus there is a suggestion that anti-dsDNA is present. Antibodies related to SLE, such as anti-dsDNA and anti-Sm, have to be looked at when there is a suspicion of this diagnostic hypothesis. In a study of 72 patients with primary Sjogren's, decreased salivary flow (according to the European classification criteria) correlated with the presence of ANA, anti-Ro/SSA, and anti-La/SSB. No such correlation was seen for the lacrimal flow, and there was no mutual correlation between lacrimal and salivary flow.

Anti-Alpha-Fodrin, Anti-Acetylcholine Muscarinic Receptor M3 Antibodies, and Other Recently Described Autoantibodies

Anti-alpha-fodrin (a 120kD extracellular matrix protein) seems to be a good candidate for the role of a major autoantigen in Sjogren's, as it was found to play an important role in the P53 knockout mouse model—it was more common in juvenile forms, its pathogenic role was suggested, and it might have a prognostic value. Anti-alpha-fodrin was not specific for Sjogren's, since it was also found in a lower frequency in patients with SLE without Sjogren's. The anti-acetylcholine muscarinic receptors inhibit muscarinic receptors on parasympathetic neurotransmission and are a new marker for diagnosis for primary and secondary Sjogren's. Autoantibodies against anti-acetylcholine muscarinic receptors may be considered among the serum factors implicated in the pathophysiology of the development of primary Sjogren's dry eye; they are related to an accelerated loss of glandular function and could be a new marker to differentiate Sjogren's dry eye from non-Sjogren's dry eye. These findings from the physiopathogenic point of view would classify Sjogren's as a type of disease process mediated by an autoantibody targeting a neurotransmitter receptor, as in myasthenia gravis. Antibodies directed to the amino-terminal fragment of alpha-fodrin were frequently detected in Sjogren's patients compared with rheumatic disease patients without Sjogren's or healthy controls (70 versus 12 percent or 4 percent; p <0.00001). These recently described autoantibodies are rapidly moving from the basic sciences lab bench to the clinical pathology laboratory, and their role will certainly develop further in the near future. They may also become new treatment targets in this era of biologic therapy.

Hormonal Changes

Hormonal changes such as prolactin elevation have been reported in up to 46 percent of the primary Sjogren's patients, more commonly in younger ones. The assessment of prolactin and other hormonal alterations in Sjogren's is crucial for proper patient handling. Prolactin is the hormone responsible for lactation stimulus; it also acts as a cellular and humoral immune modulator, mostly enhancing the immune response. Like many other proteins that act in the immune system, the gene for prolactin is encoded in the short arm of chromosome 6; it is produced in many sites, such as the pituitary gland, central nervous system cells, and lymphocytes. Its receptors are structurally similar to cytokine receptors, and there is a marked similarity in transduction pathways and signaling. Molecules structurally similar to prolactin are produced by glandular cells of Sjogren's patients, but not in controls, and are related to the presence of anti-Ro/SSA antibodies. Prolactin levels are altered in 4 to 46 percent of the patients; patient selection and study design variation account for this wide range, but as in other series, prolactin was more frequently increased in younger patients. It is of clinical interest that increased prolactin levels were related to disease activity. Thyroid autoimmune syndromes such as Graves's disease and Hashimoto's thyroiditis may coexist with Sjogren's. Primary autoimmune thyroiditis was seen in 15 percent, anti-TPO antibodies were found in 25 percent, and anti-thyroglobulin was discovered in 24 percent. ACTH and cortisol were found to have decreased basal concentration when compared to normal controls; patients also displayed a decreased response to stimulus. The female sex hormones LH, FSH, and GnRH were found to be in lower concentration when compared to normal controls.

Laboratory results may vary among different series mainly due to study design and patient population selection. But most importantly, the rheumatologist or the clinician who cares for Sjogren's patients must be aware of the methodological differences and variations in specificity and sensibility of the different laboratory techniques used. Determinations that used to be semiquantitative are quickly becoming ultrasensitive due to methodological progresses that are rapidly being adopted by clinical laboratory. This has a good side and a bad side: we are able to use some markers as disease evaluation tools, but on the other hand, some established knowledge has to change when a newer, more sensitive method replaces another one with a higher specificity. Predictors of neoplasic transformation have to be looked at with extreme care.

Labial Salivary Gland Biopsy

The expected histopathologic picture of Sjogren's is of glandular lymphocytic infiltration frequently forming lymphocytic aggregates. Salivary glands are the best tissues for histologic examination in Sjogren's, as they are affected in the majority of patients and are easily accessible for biopsy procedures. In 1966 Calman and Reifman reported for the first time the involvement of minor labial salivary glands (LSGs) in a single patient with Sjogren's. The histologic picture was similar to major salivary gland findings in patients with Sjogren's. A minor LSG biopsy is done by performing a small elliptic section in the mucous membrane of the lower lip, achieving the glandular tissue and avoiding the thin muscular layer. The procedure is done under topical anesthesia with lidocaine. The sample obtained is fixed in formalin and stained with hematoxilin/eosin. The histologic findings in earlier phases of Sjogren's are periductal and perivascular lymphocytic infiltration. The key feature for the diagnosis is the lymphocytes clusters of focal infiltrates. Specimens from non-Sjogren's patients may have scattered lymphocytes, but focal infiltrates are not characteristic. Focal lymphocytic infiltrates are evaluated according to scoring systems.

Even though salivary gland biopsy is part of the diagnostic criteria for Sjogren's, it is still a controversial procedure. The LSG biopsy has a sensitivity of 70 to 83 percent, depending on the scoring system used. Patients with Sjogren's confirmed by other tests may have normal LSG in a minority of cases. Some authors question the high specificity of the biopsy. Focal lymphocytic infiltrates were also encountered in other disorders not related to Sjogren's. Therefore, a positive LSG biopsy should be considered carefully together with clinical symptoms and diagnostic tests. In patients with symptoms of oral and ocular dryness, positive ocular tests and positive serology for anti-Ro/SSA and anti-La/SSB, LSG biopsy is probably unnecessary, as these findings are enough to establish the diagnosis. If the patient has the symptoms of oral and ocular dryness, positive ocular and oral signs, and negative serology, a biopsy would probably be helpful, because if the results are positive, the patient will meet the criteria and the diagnosis will be concluded. Nevertheless, experienced pathologists must evaluate the biopsies, and grading systems should be used. Higher scores are more specific for Sjogren's. The biopsy results must be considered along with other tests; while an LSG biopsy would be positive in 87 percent of Sjogren's cases; in some it might add little or no information.

Salivary Gland Scintigraphy

The oral component of Sjogren's may also be evaluated by salivary gland scintigraphy. Salivary gland scintigraphy is a noninvasive nuclear medicine technique for the assessment of major salivary glands. A radionuclide, pertechnetium m99, is infused intravenously; after sixty minutes images of major salivary glands are captured by a nuclear chamber and transmitted to a computer. The uptake of pertechnetium by the glands is observed as well as the amount of saliva containing the radionuclide. Measuring the uptake after salivary stimulation with lemon can complement the method; delayed or diminished uptake is suggestive of Sjogren's. Scintigraphy is a tool for the evaluation of the oral component in the European criteria for Sjogren's. It is a noninvasive, qualitative, and dynamic test and has the advantage of evaluating the four major salivary glands (bilateral parotids and submandibulary glands) simultaneously; thus it can complement labial gland biopsy, which examines only the minor salivary glands. Scintigraphy of salivary glands is highly sensitive for Sjogren's but has a low specificity. The pertechnetium uptake of m99 is frequently diminished in normal controls and in patients with other connective tissue diseases. Reduced uptake by scintigraphy correlates with reduced salivary flow by sialometry and with abnormal ocular tests. Therefore patients with diminished salivary flow on sialometry and positive rose bengal test will probably have abnormal salivary gland scintigraphy.

Summing Up

Blood testing can be very useful in diagnosing primary and secondary Sjogren's syndrome, identifying clinical subsets, and assessing inflammatory activity. Infrequently, a biopsy of tissue or imaging studies may be needed to assist in localizing or better characterizing a pathologic process.

Robert F. Spiera

Harry Spiera

13 How Can I Be Sure It's Really Sjogren's?

IN THIS CHAPTER, we will explore the differential diagnosis of Sjogren's syndrome and the occurrence of sicca (dryness) and other Sjogren's features in other, nonautoimmune conditions that can mimic Sjogren's.

It is important to be as accurate as possible in the diagnosis of Sjogren's for several reasons. At times, the clinical features being addressed may have an easily treatable alternative explanation, so diagnostic accuracy allows true resolution of the problem rather than just further management of the problem, which of course is often imperfect. The diagnosis of Sjogren's can also have prognostic implications beyond just the experienced subjective complaints, so erroneously assigning the diagnosis can burden the patient with concerns (such as the increased risk of lymphoproliferative disease) that may indeed be misplaced. Finally, Sjogren's may be mimicked by other potentially dangerous health conditions in which earlier diagnosis may allow for improved clinical outcome.

Environmental Factors

The hallmark features of Sjogren's—dryness of the eyes and mouth—can be seen in many other medical conditions (Table 13.1). Outside influences can also play a major role. Simple environmental factors such as very dry heat in the winter months might contribute to a subjective sense of dryness, but it would be unusual for that to result in complications of dryness (such as corneal abrasions or cavities) or even measurable severe dryness on objective testing such as Schirmer's testing of eye

---

TABLE 13.1 NON-AUTOIMMUNE CAUSES OF DRYNESS

Environment
Age
Medications
  • Antidepressants
  • Antipsychotics
  • Neuroleptics
  • Anticholinergics
  • Antihistamines
  • Diuretics
  • Estrogens (dry eye)
Metabolic
  • Diabetes
  • Hypothyroidism

---

moisture. Medications can be an important cause of sicca symptoms and should always be considered carefully in evaluation of the patient complaining of dryness. Antidepressants, particularly the tricyclic class, are notorious for causing dryness, particularly of the mouth, which in some individuals may be severe. These medications are used to treat not just depression but also sleep disorders and even chronic pain and therefore are widely used in the general population. Hormone replacement therapy in postmenopausal women has been shown to increase the risk of developing significant dry eye symptoms, possibly related to an effect on the quality of the tear film. Diuretics, used to treat high blood pressure and/or edema (fluid retention), can be drying, particularly when used at high doses. Often routine laboratory studies such as electrolytes can offer a clue that this side effect is manageable, and should be evaluated particularly in patients with sicca complaints being treated with these medications. Other medications that can have significant drying effects include anticholinergic medications, often used to treat bladder conditions or gastrointestinal motility disorders. Many of the antipsychotic medications used to treat psychiatric disease as well as medications used to treat Parkinson's disease similarly have significant anticholinergic effects, resulting in dryness. Antihistamines are widely used to treat allergies and are a cause of dryness. These drugs are now available over the counter, and patients therefore may not even think of including them in their list of medications when consulting a physician for evaluation. They nevertheless can be a major factor contributing to the development of sicca. Meticulous review of medications is therefore imperative in evaluating patients for the possibility of Sjogren's. Often the identified culprit can be withdrawn or another, less drying medication substituted. Moreover, even in patients with well-established Sjogren's, use of these medications may exacerbate the dryness and should be considered.

Age

Another consideration in evaluating dryness is advancing age. As people get older, there is a tendency to have less robust ocular and oral moisture, often on a degenerative rather than an autoimmune basis. Approximately one-third of elderly patients complain of significant dryness, and of course in only a minority of these is Sjogren's syndrome the culprit. Furthermore, as people age they are more likely to have a myriad of other medical problems, such as hypertension, bladder difficulties, or depression, that may be treated with the aforementioned medications. This can further exacerbate the sicca complaints, as discussed above. It is important, however, to recognize that advanced age does not preclude a diagnosis of Sjogren's, but rather should lead to some pause in making the diagnosis, particularly in the absence of serological support for the diagnosis.

Infections

A variety of infections can also cause features mimicking Sjogren's syndrome. Parotid enlargement, oral dryness, and fatigue can occur in the context of mumps infection, but in that setting it is usually a self-limiting problem. Bacterial infection of parotid glands can occur, but generally it is more of an acute illness and tends not to be confused diagnostically with Sjogren's syndrome. Tuberculosis or even leprosy, however, can be unusually infectious causes of parotitis and cause systemic symptoms such as fever and fatigue, and should be considered in the differential diagnosis in a patient who might be at risk for those infections.

HIV infection has been associated with a syndrome that appears clinically similar to Sjogren's, diffuse infiltrative lymphocytosis syndrome (DILS). Similar to primary Sjogren's patients, DILS patients can have significant sicca complaints, may demonstrate salivary gland enlargement (including both the parotid and minor salivary glands), and may have other nonspecific complaints such as joint pain and fatigue. Even biopsy of affected glands may not distinguish this syndrome from Sjogren's, as there can be a similar tissue appearance. Specialized staining of the biopsy tissue, however, shows that the immune cells infiltrating the glandular tissues are different from those that are seen in Sjogren's patients (T8 or suppressor T cells in DILS, versus T4 or helper T cells in Sjogren's syndrome). Patients with DILS and HIV are much less likely to have the typical autoantibodies of Sjogren's such as anti-Ro/SSA, anti-La/SSB, or rheumatoid factor. HIV infection should therefore be considered, particularly in patients with seronegative Sjogren's, and risk factors for HIV should be considered in anyone diagnosed with Sjogren's.

Relatively recently, hepatitis C has been recognized as the most common cause of non-A, non-B hepatitis, affecting perhaps as much as 1 percent of the population. Investigators have questioned whether hepatitis C infection may be associated with the development of Sjogren's, although studies have yielded conflicting results. There may be a subset of Sjogren's syndrome appearing in association with hepatitis C infection, although given the relatively common occurrence of hepatitis C infection in the general population, it is hard to establish cause and effect. Like patients with Sjogren's syndrome, patients with hepatitis C seem to be at increased risk for lymphoma compared to the general population. Even serologically the issue can be confusing, as patients with hepatitis C virus infection (or any chronic liver condition, for that matter) can develop positive rheumatoid factor, commonly encountered in patients with Sjogren's syndrome. In patients with fatigue, joint pain, and a positive rheumatoid factor without other supporting Sjogren's serologies such as SSA and SSB antibodies, it may be prudent to screen for hepatitis C infection, which can be done by a simple blood test.

Metabolic Disorders

Metabolic disorders may also mimic Sjogren's syndrome. Patients with diabetes often complain of excessive thirst and a subjective sense of dryness. Fatigue is also common with poorly controlled blood sugar. Other symptoms such as very frequent urination or blurred vision may help guide the physician to the more appropriate diagnosis of diabetes. Even the very most basic laboratory testing usually includes determination of blood sugar levels, and diabetes is therefore not often a hard diagnosis to make. Another endocrine disorder that can be associated with Sjogren's-like features is thyroid disease. Underactive thyroid can result in dryness of the mouth, vagina, skin, and hair. Fatigue is often a major complaint, and joint and muscle pain is common. Routine physical exam will usually reveal abnormal reflexes that might point to the diagnosis. Blood tests can confirm the diagnosis of an underactive thyroid gland but must be specifically ordered. Underactive thyroid is easily treatable; more importantly, it can be dangerous if left unrecognized and untreated. Interestingly, thyroid abnormalities are more common in patients with Sjogren's syndrome and other autoimmune diseases as well, so when there are symptoms of increasing fatigue and musculoskeletal pain, even in a patient with well-established Sjogren's, it is worthwhile to check for the presence of thyroid function test abnormalities.

Fibromyalgia and Chronic Fatigue Syndrome

Other, less well defined generalized disorders may also be confused with Sjogren's syndrome or, conversely, can complicate the course of Sjogren's syndrome. Fibromyalgia is a rheumatic disorder characterized by widespread musculoskeletal pain, often more of muscles than joints themselves, without an inflammatory or recognized autoimmune basis to the subjective complaints. Fatigue can be a prominent component of this syndrome as well. There is a strong association with poor sleep, and nonrestorative sleep is felt to be a contributing factor in the development of this syndrome. Other medications used to treat fibromyalgia have significant drying effects, including pain medications such as narcotic analgesics, or antidepressant medications, which may be used to aid sleep, to treat chronic pain, or of course to treat underlying depression, which often occurs in fibromyalgia. Hence these patients may have the constellation of symptoms—sicca features, fatigue, and pain—that often is associated with Sjogren's syndrome. Immunomodulatory interventions such as antimalarial medications or corticosteroids, however, do not help fibromyalgia patients, and therefore it is important to recognize fibromyalgia as a potential alternative cause of the symptoms in patients being evaluated for Sjogren's syndrome. Patients with fibromyalgia typically do not have the lab test abnormalities that are associated with Sjogren's syndrome. Conversely, patients with well-established Sjogren's often have disordered sleep habits related to frequent nocturnal urination (a result of increased fluid intake while awake), as well as stress and anxiety related to the underlying rheumatic disease, all of which increase their risk for developing secondary fibromyalgia. This must be considered in evaluating new complaints of pain and fatigue, even in a patient with well-established Sjogren's, so that effective therapy can be instituted or—just as important—inappropriate immunomodulatory or immunosuppressive interventions not be initiated for what is not an inflammatory or autoimmune-based constellation of symptoms.

Chronic fatigue syndrome is a related syndrome with many features that overlap with those of fibromyalgia. Patients with chronic fatigue syndrome often report that from a functional standpoint, fatigue is a more limiting feature than muscle or joint pain. Like fibromyalgia, no underlying inflammatory or autoimmune abnormality has been well defined, but questions have been raised regarding relationships to various viral infections. Mild lymph gland enlargement has been described in association with this syndrome as well, but not the robust enlargement or parotid enlargement that can be seen in Sjogren's syndrome. The symptoms tend not to respond to immunomodulatory interventions such as corticosteroids. Although chronic fatigue can be a very prominent complaint in the context of Sjogren's, fatigue alone in the absence of objective evidence of significant dryness or other serological abnormalities would argue more for the diagnosis of chronic fatigue syndrome than Sjogren's per se.

Other Autoimmune Conditions

It is recognized that there is much overlap between the various autoimmune diseases. The distinction between primary and secondary Sjogren's has been addressed in Chapter 11. Other immune-mediated conditions, however, may be associated with Sjogren's-like complaints but represent different disease entities. Sarcoidosis is an inflammatory condition that can result in parotid and other glandular enlargement, sicca symptoms, often significant eye inflammation, joint pain, and most commonly lung inflammation. Biopsies of affected tissue reveal granuloma, a different finding than would be seen in tissue specimens from patients with Sjogren's syndrome. Patients with sarcoidosis generally do not develop the autoantibodies seen in Sjogren's syndrome. Autoimmune liver disease can also be associated with Sjogren's-like features. In particular, primary biliary cirrhosis is an autoimmune liver condition with a high rate of subjective sicca complaints, joint pain, and even joint swelling as well as fatigue. Many of these patients do indeed have Sjogren's syndrome, and biopsy of salivary glands reveals changes typical of Sjogren's syndrome. Conversely, patients with Sjogren's syndrome can develop autoimmune liver disease consistent with primary biliary cirrhosis. It therefore becomes largely semantic whether we call the disorder primary Sjogren's complicated by primary biliary cirrhosis, or primary biliary cirrhosis with secondary Sjogren's syndrome. The main practical point is that chronic liver disease can be associated with Sjogren's syndrome, and that measurement of liver function tests should be included in laboratory testing of patients suspected of having Sjogren's syndrome.

Summing Up

Sjogren's syndrome refers to a constellation of clinical features that share an autoimmune basis. Many of the features, however, such as dryness, fatigue, pain, and even glandular enlargement can occur as the result of non-autoimmune conditions such as medications, age, metabolic abnormalities, or infection. These alternative explanations must be considered when making the diagnosis of Sjogren's, particularly when the typical blood test abnormalities (serologies) are not present. Just as important, in patients with well-established Sjogren's an exacerbation or change in symptoms may be related to these other nonautoimmune factors. It is vital to consider these, particularly when making therapeutic decisions.

PART IV

The Management of
Sjogren's Syndrome

There are four approaches toward treating Sjogren's syndrome. First, physical measures include exercise and attention to environmental factors such as sleep, climate, and geography. Next, since the "head bone" is connected to the "Sjogren's bone," emotional support as well as measures taken to create an optimal atmosphere to promote healing can be ameliorative. Third, medications exist that modulate the immune system or provide symptomatic treatment for symptoms such as dryness. Finally, surgical options such as biopsies may be needed under certain circumstances. This section will review how a practitioner manages patients with Sjogren's syndrome.

14 Treatment of Dry Eye

THE EYES ARE FREQUENTLY affected in Sjogren's syndrome, with dry eye one of the most common manifestations. Because vision connects us to the outside world, disruption of visual perceptions has a profound impact on our relationship to the world and our sense of well-being.

Dry eye occurs frequently in the general population. Recent studies suggest that as many as 40 million to 60 million Americans may be affected. Estimates of 3 million to 8 million patients with moderate to severe dry eye in the United States have been reported recently. Of these, about 2 million to 4 million will have Sjogren's syndrome. Chapters 4 and 6 discuss the cause and diagnosis of dry eye in great detail. A review follows as a prelude to a discussion of its management.

A Brief Review of Dry Eye

The most common symptoms associated with dry eye involve discomfort—sensations of dryness, irritation, itching, burning, a foreign body in the eye, grittiness, or sandiness. In addition, it is now known that symptoms of eye fatigue, which are common in Sjogren's, are probably related to problems maintaining clear vision between blinks. In an unconscious attempt to maintain a smooth tear film there is a tendency to blink more frequently; over time this causes ocular fatigue. While only a small percentage of patients with Sjogren's have dryness severe enough to threaten permanent visual loss, it is important to have an ophthalmologic examination with an initial diagnosis and periodic follow-up examinations.

Diagnosis of Dry Eye

The ophthalmologist will perform a complete eye examination, which will include a measure of vision both with and without correction (glasses or contact lenses) and an examination of the front part of the eye using a special microscope called a slit lamp. This enables the doctor to check the surface of the eye, the lids and tear glands, and the interior of the eye up to the lens (the location of cataracts). Further tests include an exam of the retina and vitreous humor, which occupy the back of the eye. This exam usually requires the use of dilating drops, which allow for a full view of retinal tissue.

In addition, other tests may be performed. In patients complaining of ocular irritation and suspected of having dry eye, a Schirmer test is commonly performed. This involves a small strip of filter paper folded over the lower lid, inserted into the tear film, and left in place for five minutes. The length of the strip that is wetted is a measure of the amount of tears present. Other tests may include the instillation of special dyes into the eye (rose bengal, lissamine green, fluorescein). These dyes stain surface cells damaged from dryness or inflammation. Abnormal instability of the tear film is a hallmark of dry eye; this is measured by the tear film breakup test. A small amount of fluorescein dye is instilled in the tears to help visualize them. Using a special filter in the slit lamp that lights up the fluorescein, the doctor can measure how rapidly the tear film is breaking up. Some doctors also use this dye to estimate how rapidly tears are exiting into the drainage pathways (tear clearance test); this is a reflection of how rapidly new tears are being produced. New research is under way to develop a simple, reliable tests (e.g., tear lysozyme, tear lactoferrin, tear osmolarity) that will provide additional information on ocular surface conditions and be suitable for widespread use in clinics and physicians' offices.

Treatment of Dry Eye

The use of *artificial tears* to supplement natural tear production and replace tears lost to evaporation has been the mainstay of treatment of dry eye (Table 14.1). These products are available without prescription at pharmacies. All of them contain water, salts, polymers (thickening agents), stabilizers, and pH buffers. In addition, many of the tear substitutes contain preservatives to protect against infection. Unfortunately, most preservatives used in artificial tear solutions are toxic to the surface of the eye when used more than four times a day. Over the last decade most companies have introduced tear substitutes without preservatives; these products are packaged in small, one-time-use dispensers, and once

TABLE 14.1 ARTIFICIAL TEAR PREPARATIONS

Major Component(s)	Concentration (%)	Trade Name	Preservative/EDTA*
Carboxymethyl cellulose	0.5%	Refresh Plus	None
		Refresh Tears	Purite
	1%	Celluvisc	None
	0.25%	Theratears	None
Glycerin	0.3%	Moisture Eyes	Benzalkonium chloride
			Benzalkonium chloride, EDTA
	1.0%	Computer Eye Drops	
Hydroxyprophyl cellulose	5 mg/insert	Lacrisert (biodegradable insert)	None
Hydroxypropyl methylcellulose	0.2%–0.3%	GenTeal	Sodium perborate
		GenTeal Gel	Sodium perborate
		GenTeal Mild	Sodium perborate
	0.5%	Tearisol	Benzalkonium chloride, EDTA
Hydroxypropyl methylcellulose, dextran 70		Blon Tears	None
		Lacritears	Benzalkonium chloride, EDTA
			Benzalkonium chloride, EDTA
		Tears Renewed	
Hydroxypropyl methylcellulose, glycerin		Clear Eyes CLR	Sorbic acid, EDTA
		Visine for Contacts	Potassium sorbate, EDTA
Hydroxypropyl methylcellulose, glycerin, dextran 70		Tears Naturale Forte	Polyquad
		Tears Naturale Free	None
Hydroxypropyl methylcellulose, glycerin, PEG-400		Visine Tears	Benzalkonium chloride
			None
		Visine Preservative Free	
Methylcellulose	1%	Murocel	Methyl-, propylparabens
Polycarbophll, PEG-400, dextran 70		AquaSite	EDTA
		AquaSite multi-dose	EDTA, Sorbic acid
Polyvinyl alcohol	1.4%	AKWA Tears	Benzalkonium chloride, EDTA
Polyvinyl alcohol, PEG-400, dextrose	1%	HypoTears	Benzalkonium chloride, EDTA
			EDTA
		HypoTears PF	
Polyvinyl alcohol, povidone	1.4%	Murine Tears	Benzalkonium chloride, EDTA

*EDTA = ethylenediaminetetraacetic acid.

TABLE 14.2   OCULAR LUBRICANTS

---

1. Lanolin-free products
   Ointments: Hypotears, Moisture Eyes PM, Puralube, Tears Renewed
   Gel: Gen Teal
2. Lanolin-containing products
   Ointments: Artificial Tears, Akwa tears, Dry Eyes, Duratears Naturale,
       Lacrilube NP, Lacrilube SOP, Lubritears, Refresh PM

---

the seal is broken they should not be used again. Tear substitutes provide moisture to the eye and increase lubrication between the lids and the surface of the eye. The major limitation of artificial tears is their short duration of action. Nonetheless, they provide relief for most patients suffering from dry eye. Several new products contain ingredients that limit tear evaporation or stabilize the tear film. Ocular lubricants are usually applied at bedtime (see Table 14.2). For more information see Appendix 3.

Punctal occlusion involves closing of the tear drainage openings located at the inner edges of the lids. This can be accomplished by inserting a small plug that blocks the outflow of tears and serves to thicken the tear film. Punctal plugs are either temporary (they dissolve) or permanent (that is, they do not dissolve, but they can become dislodged). Alternatively, permanent blockage of the outflow channels can be accomplished by applying heat or laser energy to the openings (punctual cautery); this causes a scar to form. These measures work well for most patients with dry eye. Care, however, should be exercised to make sure tear production is low enough that blocking of tear outflow will not cause epiphoria (an overflow of tears onto the face). This can be very disconcerting.

Many patients with dry eye have *blepharitis,* which is also known as Meibomian gland dysfunction. The dysfunction of these glands located at the edges of the eyelids causes excessive tear evaporation and dryness. Treatments directed to improving the function of these important glands include the application of hot compresses to the lids and cleansing of the lid margins with a moist cloth and/or a cotton-tipped applicator. In addition, the use of broad-spectrum antibiotic such as tetracycline or minocycline, taken by mouth, can provide considerable relief from symptoms.

Another area that excited a great deal of interest recently is the use of *nutritional supplements* to treat dry eye. Specifically, there is reason to believe that the ingestion of foods or nutritional supplements containing omega-3 and omega-6 essential fatty acids can aid in the synthesis of the oils produced by the Meibomian glands of the lid. These essential fatty acids are found in flaxseed oil, fish oils, and in supplements found in pharmacies, natural food stores, and supermarkets. While no large, controlled studies have yet been published, there is considerable anecdotal evidence from patients and physicians to support their value.

Recently the Food and Drug Administration approved the first prescription drop therapeutic treatment for dry eye directed to improving cell function rather than treating a symptom. This medication, cyclosporin A (Restasis, Allergan), suppresses inflammation in the eye tissue and allows the glands to recover their function. It must be taken for at least three to six months before significant improvement can be seen, and not all patients respond. How long treatment must be maintained has not yet been determined.

Currently, no FDA-approved drugs are available for tear stimulation. However, data from clinical studies also suggest that medication used to treat dry mouth (e.g., pilocarpine) may also provide symptomatic relief of dry eye.

A number of other approaches to the treatment of dry eye are currently in clinical testing. These include medications that stimulate production of mucin by the surface cells of the eye; medications that supply hormones to the glands of the eye, restoring the balance important for glandular function; agents that stabilize the tear film; and others that suppress inflammation. In the not too distant future it is likely that your doctor will have an increasing variety of new treatments to relieve pain and restore the eye tissue to a more normal state.

Special Considerations

Patients with dry eye who also have other eye problems necessitating surgery, such as cataracts, should know that there is a slightly increased risk for delayed healing after surgery. This is usually not a serious problem, and patients can anticipate equally good results. They should, however, discuss their dry eye with their surgeon, since it might necessitate a slight change in surgical technique or medication schedule. Patients who wish to undergo Lasik surgery should discuss the pros and cons of the procedure with their rheumatologist and ophthalmologist.

Patients and Their Environment

Patients with dry eye are highly sensitive to the environment. Dry and/or windy conditions—such as on an airplane or when biking—promote loss of tears through evaporation. The frequent instillation of artificial tears when in these situations can prove remarkably successful in alleviating irritative symptoms. In addition, prolonged use of video terminals decreases the frequency of blinking, thus causing excessive tear loss. Studies have shown that lowering the computer monitor below eye level results in a decrease in the width of the eyelid opening and significantly conserves tears.

The use of wraparound glasses or side panels with spectacles (moisture chamber glasses) can limit the effects of air currents on tear evaporation. The use of cool compresses during periods of ocular irritation can provide relief. The secret is to experiment with these techniques, use tear substitutes and other treatments prescribed by the doctor, and adjust activities to minimize environmental challenges. Most patients can experience considerable improvement and enhance their sense of well-being. The future is promising for continued development of even better treatments.

Summing Up

Dry eye in Sjogren's is managed with artificial tears, punctal occlusion, ocular lubricants, cyclosporine drops, or possibly dietary or environmental measures. In clinical development are exciting new agents that will change the way we approach dry eye in the next few years.

Philip C. Fox, DDS

15 Treatment of Dry Mouth

DRY MOUTH IS A hallmark symptom of Sjogren's syndrome. The term *xerostomia* is used in the medical literature to describe this subjective sensation of dryness of the oral cavity. The cause of dry mouth in Sjogren's syndrome is a reduction in the amount of saliva produced by the major and minor salivary glands and changes in the composition of the secretions. This is a result of autoimmune-mediated alterations in the salivary glands that lead to a loss of fluid-secreting cells and disruption of normal secretion mechanisms.

A Brief Review of Dry Mouth

There are three pairs of major salivary glands—the parotid, submandibular, and sublingual glands—and hundreds of minor salivary glands scattered throughout the oral cavity. These glands produce and secrete into the mouth a complex fluid containing critical protective factors. Saliva helps preserve the dentition, protect the oral soft tissues, and facilitate important oral functions such as chewing, swallowing, and speaking. In the absence of adequate salivation, there are many negative effects in the mouth. Due to the loss of the antimicrobial, remineralizing, and cleansing properties of saliva, there is a marked increase in dental caries. Caries may appear and progress rapidly. Microbial populations are altered in the mouth, resulting in an increased incidence of bacterial and fungal infections. In particular, candida infections are frequent and may be resistant to treatment. The oral mucosa may become thinner, reddened, and painful, with sensitivity to spicy foods. Chewing and swallowing become more difficult with less fluid present in the mouth. It may be hard to form a compact food bolus and move it through the oral cavity to the pharynx. Speaking may be compromised due to lack of lubrication of the soft tissues. Even taste may be affected, as tastants must be in solution in order to be fully appreciated. Accompanying these changes is a persistent feeling of dryness, not just of the mouth, but also of the throat, nose, and pharynx. The salivary gland dysfunction of Sjogren's syndrome has profound effects on the oral cavity and oral functions.

Treatment of Dry Mouth

Simple relief of symptoms of oral dryness is desirable but incomplete. There are several goals to treatment of salivary gland dysfunction and xerostomia in Sjogren's syndrome: (1) to relieve dryness symptoms, (2) to prevent anticipated oral complications, (3) to stimulate salivary gland function, and (4) to promote repair of salivary gland damage. The ideal therapy would accomplish all these. At present, however, there is no single treatment that will satisfy all these goals. However, with careful attention, close cooperation between patients and professionals, and a systematic approach to treatment, most aspects of dry mouth in Sjogren's syndrome can be managed and improved.

The mainstay of symptomatic treatment is water. The importance of *adequate hydration* of the oral cavity for the Sjogren's syndrome patient cannot be overemphasized. Water should always be available, with small sips taken frequently. Water does more than relieve the immediate sense of dryness. It helps hydrate the oral mucosa and cleanse the mouth, partially replacing these functions of saliva. Dehydration causes oral dryness and reduced salivary output, so adequate water intake is important to maintain maximum salivary function. If small amounts of water are used each time, this will limit the total volume consumed and reduce frequent urination, a complaint of many patients. Small sips of water also help chewing and swallowing.

Increasing the humidity may be helpful as well. During the winter months, humidity can be very low, and this will contribute to feelings of oral dryness. This is a particular problem at night, when salivary function normally is reduced and breathing is often through the mouth. The use of a humidifier placed at the bedside can help relieve nighttime dryness, thereby improving sleep. Humidifiers should be cleaned often and the water in the reservoir replaced daily.

There are many saliva replacement products (see Appendix 3). Patients should try different products to see if any are beneficial. The effects are temporary but may be helpful for those with very dry mouth. In Europe, there are saliva replacement products that contain mucins (a prominent component of human saliva) from animal sources. These are reported to have greater patient acceptance, but the studies are limited. Some patients use artificial saliva at bedtime and during the night in order to limit their nighttime water intake and the subsequent need for frequent urination during the night.

There are also numerous *moisturizers, lubricants, rinses, gels,* and *emollients* (see Appendix 3) that are promoted for relief of dry mouth symptoms. These can be applied to the lips and inside of the mouth. Personal preference should guide the selection of a product. Most will provide temporary relief of dryness and mucosal discomfort. Alcohol, tobacco and caffeine can have drying effects on the oral cavity and should be avoided or limited. Many carbonated beverages contain caffeine and are quite acidic. They should not be used regularly for relief of dryness symptoms.

Symptoms often can be relieved effectively by stimulating salivary output. Means of doing this are discussed below in the section on stimulation of salivary gland function.

Prevention of Oral Complications

Generation of *dental caries* requires the presence of bacteria and a carbohydrate source for them to metabolize. Therefore, much of the destruction of the teeth found in Sjogren's syndrome patients can be controlled with vigorous oral hygiene measures and dietary modifications. Meticulous oral hygiene should include flossing at least daily and tooth brushing after each meal. The goal is to remove the bacteria that attach to the teeth, as well as their food sources. In the absence of cariogenic bacteria, decay will not occur. Similarly, if the bacteria are deprived of fermentable carbohydrates, they will not produce acids that can demineralize the tooth surface. Sugar in the diet should be minimized, and sticky sweets, such as cookies and candies that adhere to the teeth, should be avoided. When sugary foods are consumed, the teeth should be brushed—or at least rinsed—immediately. Regular use of acidic beverages, like many soft drinks, should be avoided as well. In addition to oral hygiene and diet, the use of fluoride is an important preventive measure. Fluoride helps to repair early demineralization of the tooth (the first step in dental caries) and strengthens the tooth surface. A fluoride-containing toothpaste should be used, and topical fluoride applications may be indicated. The frequency, type, and mode of application of topical fluoride (daily, weekly; rinse, high-concentration gel; self- or professionally applied; brushed on, applied in a custom tray, etc.) should be discussed with the dentist. The determination should be made based on the caries rate and severity of the salivary gland dysfunction. In some cases, a fluoride varnish may be applied to the teeth by the dentist. Experimental studies have shown that early caries can be repaired with solutions containing high concentrations of calcium and phosphate. This is one of the prominent functions of natural saliva. The use of a remineralizing solution may be indicated in Sjogren's syndrome patients and should be discussed with the dentist.

Fungal infections, usually caused by *Candida albicans* spp., are common in dry mouth patients. A confusing aspect of diagnosis is that these often do not present in the common white mucocutaneous form (known by most people as "thrush"). Instead, the mucosa may appear red or irritated, the so-called chronic erythematous form of candidiasis. Patients may complain of a burning sensation. The area should be cultured and treatment instituted with a topical therapeutic. Due to a lack of natural antifungal components usually provided in saliva, the infection may recur. Many infections are difficult to manage and resistant to therapy, and treatment may be prolonged. This is a problem, as most topical antifungal preparations (rinses and lozenges) have a very high sugar content. A rinse without sugar should be used or formulated. If a sugar-containing preparation is used, particularly a slowly dissolving lozenge, patients must brush well afterward. Although use of a systemic antifungal agent seems ideal in Sjogren's syndrome, if salivary function is low this approach may also fail, as much of the drug is delivered through salivary secretion and may fail to reach the affected mucosa. Aggressive topical treatment will be successful given sufficient time and may be repeated as often as necessary.

**TABLE 15.1   MEANS OF STIMULATING
SALIVARY FUNCTION**

Topical/Local Approaches

   Gustatory stimulation
   Masticatory stimulation
   Anhydrous crystalline maltose
   Acupuncture

Systemic Secretogogues

   Pilocarpine
   Cevimeline
   Bromhexine
   Anetholetrithione
   TNF-alpha blockers

Stimulation of Salivary Function

There are many ways to stimulate salivary output. They may be divided into topical or local approaches and systemic therapies (Table 15.1). By stimulating the remaining salivary gland tissue, a patient will get all the benefits of natural saliva in the oral cavity and relief of dryness symptoms. The success of this is dependent on the amount of secretory function that remains and the efficacy of the stimulation. Even modest increases in salivary output may translate into significant symptomatic improvement. A deficiency in all current therapies is the transient nature of the stimulation. Even systemic parasympathomimetic drugs have a duration of action of only a few hours. However, symptomatic relief of dryness may persist beyond the immediate period of increased salivary output with chronic use of these agents. This is likely due to beneficial effects on the mucosa from the increased amounts of saliva.

Topical and Local Therapies

Saliva can be stimulated effectively by almost any oral activity. Chewing or sucking on an object will result in a robust increase in saliva output. Salivation is also responsive to taste, particularly sour and bitter. The use of *flavored gums and lozenges* remains a mainstay of palliative therapy of dry mouth. The combination of gustatory and masticatory stimulation can transiently increase salivation and relieve symptoms of dry mouth. Patients with diminished salivation should use sugar-free gums, lozenges, candies, or mints for symptomatic relief of xerostomia. The use of sugar-free products must be stressed, as otherwise the addition of sugar bathing the dentition will only increase the caries risk and negate the benefits of increased salivary output. Xylitol is an acceptable sweetener that has been shown to reduce dental caries. Recent clinical trials have reported on the use of a lozenge composed of anhydrous crystalline maltose as a treatment for dry mouth in Sjogren's syndrome. Maltose has a very low cariogenic potential and may improve symptoms and salivary function. Some patients benefit from sucking on a cherry pit, smooth stone, or other non-nutritive object. This may increase salivation without any sugar or calories.

Although not strictly a local therapy, *acupuncture* relies on application of the needles to specific locations, often in close proximity to the oral cavity. There have been a number of clinical studies of acupuncture to treat xerostomia, and the authors reported some benefit for relief of symptoms and improvement in salivary output. One problem with these studies is the difficulty in providing for appropriate placebo controls in clinical trials of acupuncture. One trial that used superficial, non-site-specific acupuncture as a control found that the control group had improvements similar to those of the active acupuncture group. At present, acupuncture remains a possible approach to enhancing salivary function that requires further study. Acupuncture may serve as a useful adjunct to management of dry mouth.

Systemic Therapies

There are many systemic agents that are capable of stimulating salivary output (Table 15.1). The most extensive clinical evidence has been with pilocarpine (Salagen). Pilocarpine is a parasympathomimetic agent with mild beta-adrenergic-stimulating properties. It has been proposed as a treatment for dry mouth for over a hundred years. A number of well-designed and well-controlled studies of substantial size have examined the effects of pilocarpine on dry mouth and salivary function in patients with Sjogren's syndrome. These clinical trials have consistently demonstrated that at doses of 5 to 10 mg three or four times daily (maximum 30 mg a day), pilocarpine can significantly improve symptoms of dry mouth and increase salivary output. Salivary secretion is maximally stimulated approximately one hour after dosing with pilocarpine, and increases over baseline salivary output are found for three to four hours. No tolerance to the secretogogue effects of pilocarpine has been reported, nor has long-term improvement in baseline salivary function been found. Increased salivary output is transient, dose-related, and consistent.

Serious adverse events are rare with pilocarpine. While side effects such as sweating, flushing, and urinary frequency are common, they are typically of mild or moderate intensity and of relatively short duration. Side effects may also be alleviated by taking the medication after meals. Use of pilocarpine is contraindicated in individuals with uncontrolled asthma, narrow-angle glaucoma, or acute iritis. Caution is advised with use in patients with cardiovascular disease.

Another parasympathomimetic agent, *cevimeline* (Evoxac), has also been studied in large, well-controlled trials. At doses of 30 mg three times daily, cevimeline was shown to significantly improve symptoms of dry mouth and increase salivary output in patients with Sjogren's syndrome. Cevimeline is similar pharmacologically to pilocarpine, although the onset of increased salivation may be somewhat later and the duration of action longer. The safety and adverse event profiles are very similar to pilocarpine as well, with sweating, light-headedness, and nausea common complaints among patients. Cevimeline has been reported to have a high selective affinity for M3 subtype muscarinic receptors, the predominant receptor subtype in the salivary glands.

Bromhexine, although not FDA-approved, has been proposed as a salivary stimulant and treatment for dry mouth in Sjogren's syndrome. However, there are no well-controlled studies demonstrating that this agent will increase salivary output or improve dry mouth symptoms. There may be some benefit for dry eye symptoms in Sjogren's syndrome, but this has not been shown for the oral cavity.

Anetholetrithione, although not FDA-approved, is an agent that has been demonstrated to increase salivation in individuals with mild salivary gland dysfunction. The dose studied was 25 mg three times daily. In more severe cases of secretory hypofunction in Sjogren's syndrome patients, however, anetholetrithione was ineffective. Though there has been an interesting report suggesting a synergistic effect between anetholetrithione and pilocarpine, there are inadequate clinical trials of this drug.

Several large clinical trials have been conducted using *interferon-alpha* (IFN-alpha) (not FDA-approved), as a high-dose injectable or a low-dose lozenge, for treatment of dry mouth and decreased salivation in Sjogren's syndrome. The low-dose lozenge formulation, at 150 IU three times a day, was found to reduce xerostomia and increase salivary output in some studies. In one study, after six months of treatment minor salivary gland inflammation also improved. Side effects and adverse events were minimal. Further clinical trials will be necessary to define appropriate doses and to demonstrate fully the efficacy of this experimental agent.

Infliximab, etanercept, and adalimumab are TNF-alpha blockers used in treatment of rheumatoid arthritis. (TNF-alpha is a cytokine that is felt to be a central component of inflammatory reactions.) In preliminary uncontrolled studies in Sjogren's syndrome, infliximab has shown significant benefit in a number of clinical and functional parameters, including increased salivary flow rate and improvement in symptoms of oral dryness. Some of these benefits remained after one year. A recent European multicenter placebo-controlled trial of infliximab failed to demonstrate improvement in dry mouth symptoms or salivary function compared to placebo. These disparate results need to be resolved with larger placebo-controlled studies.

Many other agents have been proposed as potential salivary stimulants and dry mouth treatments in Sjogren's syndrome. While some may be effective, there are inadequate well-controlled clinical trials available at present to recommend their use. In deciding whether to try one of these agents, it is important to look closely at the potential adverse effects and carefully consider the risk-to-benefit ratio.

Repair of Salivary Gland Alterations

There are no agents that have been shown definitively to promote repair of salivary gland damage in Sjogren's syndrome. As noted above, IFN-alpha did show improvements in minor salivary gland histopathology, although this study was in a small number of subjects and should be repeated. This is a significant finding, however, as other agents, including prednisone and a nonsteroidal anti-inflammatory drug, failed to have any effect on salivary pathology in earlier trials. Additional clinical trials that look microscopically at the salivary glands to determine the effects of the newer biologics that are being studied at present in Sjogren's syndrome, such as infliximab and etanercept, are needed.

Future Directions for Management of Dry Mouth in Sjögren's Syndrome

There is a need for improved secretogogues that will have fewer side effects, an increased duration of stimulatory activity, and greater potency. Current therapies are restricted to agents that act primarily via the muscarinic receptor. Future drugs may be directed to other receptors known to stimulate salivary cells. It is also possible that small-molecule drugs may be developed that target salivary receptors with greater specificity and consequently have fewer adverse effects.

Novel approaches will have to be found for individuals with too little remaining salivary function to be helped by approaches directed at increasing salivary output. In these individuals, directed cell growth and repair may be possible, perhaps using gene therapy techniques. This will be feasible with improved knowledge of salivary cell growth control. The goal would be natural repair of the salivary gland. There is also the possibility of salivary transplantation or creation of a biocompatible artificial salivary gland. It is likely that a combination of these approaches will result in many more therapeutic options in the near future.

Summing Up

The current management of the dry mouth is mostly symptomatic and transiently ameliorative. Medications are modestly effective but do little about the underlying process. Exciting investigations are ongoing which might lead to more definitive relief of this uncomfortable feature of the syndrome.

Aikaterini D. Chrysochou, MD

Fotini C. Soliotis, MD

Stuart S. Kassan, MD

Haralampos M. Moutsopoulos, MD

16 Systemic Therapies in Sjogren's

A MAJOR GOAL OF therapy in Sjogren's syndrome is to treat the main symptoms of dry eye and dry mouth. Replacement of decreased secretions and administration of stimulators of tear and saliva secretion are the most important therapeutic measures for those patients. In addition, a variety of drugs for specific symptoms or complications of Sjogren's are available for extraglandular involvement. Immunosuppressive therapies are reserved only for serious and life-threatening major organ involvement.

The Respiratory Tract

Sjogren's patients may also develop inflammation of the upper airways (laryngotracheobronchitis) due to dryness and difficulty handling thickened secretions. Thus mucolytic agents (e.g., guaifenesin), which reduce the viscosity of the mucus, are useful for thinning secretions of the air tubes. These agents also improve the difficulty in clearing foreign material that has been inhaled into the respiratory tract. For example, bromhexine (not available in the United States) at a dose of 48 mg/day may be of benefit. Its side effects are nausea, an unpleasant sensation that is vaguely referred to the stomach and abdomen and which often leads to vomiting, diarrhea, gastrointestinal bleeding, and rash. It is contraindicated in pregnancy, in patients with a history of peptic ulcer, and in those with active tuberculosis. Ambroxol (also not available in the United States) at a dose of 120 mg/day may also be useful in mouth and lung dryness. It should not be administered in pregnancy or during lactation, or in people suffering from peptic ulcer. Drinking a lot of water while taking these drugs should be always encouraged. Home humidifiers to moisten the air can also be of help in relieving the symptoms of mild inflammation of the air tubes (tracheobronchitis). Prescribed nebulizers that deliver water droplets into the small airways may be of some benefit. If pulmonary function tests confirm blockage of airflow in the bronchi or if wheezing is present due to very thick mucus, bronchodilators can be prescribed in combination with mucolytic drugs. Salbutamol (albuterol) relaxes smooth muscle of the small air tubes (bronchi) by action on beta-2 receptors with little effect on the heart rate. When inhaled, the usual dose is 200–400 mcg every four to six hours. The patient may experience nervousness, dizziness, fatigue, dry mouth, unpleasant taste, stomach upset, difficulty urinating, vision changes, chest pain or palpitations, muscle cramping, or tremor. Caution must be taken in patients with coronary heart disease and palpitations because beta-2 agonists can affect the heart rate. Concurrent use of beta-adrenergic blockers, such as propanolol, should be avoided because they antagonize albuterol's effects.

Inflammation of the substance of the lung (interstitial lung disease, ILD) may also occur in Sjogren's patients. The standard treatment for ILD is oral prednisone at a dose of 1 mg/kg daily with subsequent dose decrease. Prednisone is administered for at least six months, and the response is monitored with comprehensive clinical evaluation, repeated pulmonary function tests, and high-resolution lung computed tomography scans. The long-term use of corticosteroids may cause skin thinning, acne, hirsutism, cataracts, premature atherosclerosis, gastritis, peptic ulcer, menstrual disturbances, osteoporosis, muscle weakness, diabetes mellitus, hypertension, and heightened risk of infections. Patients should be careful with salt and sugar intake, may need to take medicine to minimize the risk of gastrointestinal disturbances, and should be encouraged to drink milk and to take calcium supplements and other special drugs to prevent osteoporosis. Blood tests should be done regularly in order to measure the levels of glucose and electrolytes. Steroids become less effective when co-administered with phenytoin and phenobarbital, both drugs used for epilepsy, and rifampicin, an antibiotic. They should not be given with alcohol and nonsteroidal anti-inflammatory drugs (NSAIDs), because they may induce peptic ulcer disease more easily. They also interact with digitalis (e.g., digoxin, digitoxin), some diuretics, and anticoagulants.

Azathioprine is an immunosuppressive drug that can be used as an alternative when high doses of corticosteroids are needed to control the disease. It is administered orally, at a dose of 1–2 mg/kg, usually in association with prednisone, to every symptomatic patient with ILD or those patients with functional, radiologic, or histologic evidence of ongoing interstitial lung disease. Its major side effect is myelosuppression, or toxicity in the bone marrow, which may result in decreased production of blood cells, thus making the patient susceptible to infection and bleeding. Gastrointestinal side effects occur frequently with azathioprine and are mostly loss of appetite, nausea, vomiting, and elevation of liver enzymes; monitoring of blood cells and liver function tests are necessary for these patients. Caution must also be taken that azathioprine is not administered with allopurinol, a drug used for decreasing the levels of uric acid in the blood in patients with a history of gout, because then bone marrow toxicity increases dramatically.

Other immunosuppressive drugs such as cyclophosphamide (Cytoxan) and cyclosporine (Neoral) are sometimes employed in cases resistant to the drug treatment mentioned above.

Inflammation of the pleura, the lining around the lung, is treated with nonsteroidal anti-inflammatory drugs or corticosteroids. Increased pressure in the main vessel that takes blood from the heart to the lungs (pulmonary hypertension, PHT) is a very rare complication in Sjogren's patients. PHT may occur as a result of long-standing inflammation of the lungs (ILD). Thus treatment of the underlying disease may improve pulmonary hypertension. These patients usually need oxygen therapy. Almitrine bismesylate improves oxygenation of the lungs, probably by reducing blood supply to areas of the lungs that are not well ventilated. Vasodilators such as nifedipine, hydralazine, and verapamil alleviate symptoms but do not prolong life expectancy in patients with pulmonary hypertension; they may also cause low blood pressure and faintness (hypotension), especially in association with other drugs such as beta-blockers, and increase heart rate, and so should be prescribed with caution in patients suffering from coronary heart disease.

Long-term therapy with intravenous infusion of epoprostenol (prostacycline) at an initial dose of 2 ng/kg/min is of benefit and improves life expectancy in patients with PHT. It is capable of dilating blood vessels and potentially prevents platelets from sticking together. It causes lowering of the blood pressure, and this may be worsened by other vasodilator drugs and diuretics. Risk of bleeding may be increased when co-administered with aspirin, warfarin, or heparin, which inhibit blood clotting. During therapy, patients may experience mild or severe headache, nausea, vomiting, muscle pain, back pain, difficulty in breathing, flushing, fever or chills, unusual bleeding or bruising, or diarrhea.

Thinning of the blood with warfarin to prevent blood clotting in the vessels is also effective therapy in PTH. An endothelin receptor antagonist, bosentan, is a promising new drug for the treatment of pulmonary hypertension and is administered orally. High concentrations of a substance called endothelin-1 have been found in the lungs of both primary and secondary pulmonary hypertension patients. Endothelin-1 causes vessels to become narrow and increases the thickness of the blood vessel wall. Bosentan has be shown to be of benefit in patients with pulmonary hypertension.

Kidneys

When kidneys are involved in Sjogren's patients and cannot get rid of acids (distal renal tubular acidosis, RTA), there is increased risk of kidney stone formation. Oral alkaline preparations containing sodium and potassium citrate are used to decrease this risk. Furthermore, low blood potassium level (hypokalemia) is another complication of RTA. It is usually asymptomatic but in some instances may lead to muscle weakness or even paralysis and palpitations. Increasing the intake of potassium-rich foods (such as oranges and bananas) is usually not enough on its own to raise potassium levels adequately. Intravenous administration of potassium is necessary when the potassium level is very low, while in other instances oral potassium supplements are used. The use of potassium-sparing diuretics such as amiloride, triamterene, and spironolactone is preferable in these patients. Amiloride is preferred to spironolactone because the latter can sometimes cause disturbances in the menstrual cycle in women and gynecomastia in men.

Polydipsia and polyuria due to nephrogenic diabetes insipidus (DI) is another manifestation of impaired tubular function in Sjogren's. This results from partial or complete resistance to the effects of antidiuretic hormone (ADH) in the kidney tubules. ADH is a substance produced by the brain that acts on the kidneys and normally prevents water loss. A number of therapies are available that can prevent water loss in these patients, including diuretics, NSAIDs, and a low-salt, low-protein diet.

Thiazide diuretics in combination with a low-salt diet can decrease polyuria; hydrochlorothiazide at a dose of 25 mg once or twice daily causes mild water loss from the body, diminishing water delivery to the areas of the kidney that are sensitive to ADH and thus reducing urine output. The potassium-sparing diuretic amiloride may also be helpful when administered together with thiazide diuretics because it partially blocks the potassium wasting induced by those diuretics.

NSAIDs can also be used as treatment because they enhance the action of ADH. Thus they are capable of increasing the concentrating ability of kidneys. However, not all NSAIDs have the same effect.

A low-salt, low-protein diet may also result in decreasing the urine output.

Because most patients with nephrogenic DI have partial rather than complete resistance to ADH, it is possible that bringing hormone levels above normal may increase the renal effect of ADH and reduce water loss. Therefore, desmopressin (brand name DDAVP), a drug that enhances reabsorption of water in the kidneys by increasing permeability of the collecting tubules, may be tried in patients who have polyuria refractory to the treatments mentioned above.

Glomerulonephritis, or inflammation of the kidney glomeruli, can be treated with corticosteroids and other immunosuppressive drugs. It is rare in patients with primary Sjogren's but occurs more frequently in those with other overlapping conditions and especially in systemic lupus erythematosus. The treatment of moderate to severe glomerulonephritis is high doses of corticosteroids together with another drug called cyclophosphamide given intravenously (1 g/m^2 every month for at least six months). Cyclophosphamide is an agent that prevents cell division by inhibiting DNA synthesis; it also suppresses the immune system. Because it is broken down in the liver and can affect liver function, monitoring of liver function is necessary. Another serious side effect is inflammation of the bladder, known as hemorrhagic cystitis, which may be prevented if cyclophosphamide is used in combination with a drug called mesna. A small percentage of patients may develop bladder cancer after many years of cyclophosphamide therapy. Examination of the bladder with the help of a tube (cystoscopy) may by useful for early diagnosis. Side effects of cyclophosphamide closely related to the time of infusion are headache, skin rash, facial flushing, nasal congestion, nausea and vomiting. About ten days after the infusion low counts of white cells in the blood (leucopenia) may be observed. Therefore, monitoring parameters for all patients should include a complete blood count, as well as blood urea nitrogen, uric acid, serum electrolytes, and serum creatinine before each infusion. Cyclophosphamide may decrease digoxin serum levels when co-administered, while other drugs such as allopurinol and chloramphenicol can increase its toxicity. It also interacts with anesthetic agents as well as cimetidine, doxorubicin, and thiazide diuretics. Patients must not become pregnant or breast-feed during therapy. Cyclophosphamide may induce disturbances in the menstrual cycle and even menopause, especially when administered in women over 32 years of age.

An alternative therapy is mycophenolate mofetil (2 g/day). It also suppresses the immune system, and its main side effects are nausea, vomiting, diarrhea or constipation and cramps. It may also cause blood disturbances such as low counts of white and red blood cells.

When patients with glomerulonephritis have a condition called mixed cryoglobulinemia (due to the presence of cryoglobulins, special antibodies in blood that become active in low temperature), plasmapheresis to remove the cryoglobulins may be a useful therapy.

The Gastrointestinal Tract

In addition to salivary glands, Sjogren's can affect the esophagus, the stomach, and the pancreas.

Pilocarpine is a drug commonly used for the treatment of dry mouth (xerostomia) and dry eye. It is given at a dose of 5 mg three or four times a day, and the total daily dose should not exceed 30 mg. First used for the treatment of simple chronic glaucoma, it stimulates cholinergic receptors present in the eye, the blood vessels, the heart, the lungs and the salivary glands, and as a result increases tear and saliva secretion. Side effects include sweats, flushing, feeling hot, exacerbation of asthma, and blurred vision, especially at night. Also, because it increases bowel and bladder motility, many patients need to go to the toilet frequently. In case patients do not tolerate the drug, smaller doses may be administered; for example, one to three 5 mg doses per day can be given after meals. Pilocarpine should not be administered to patients with closed-angle glaucoma or uncontrolled asthma, or in pregnancy. Its administration could potentially cause excessive slowing of the heart rate (heart block) in patients also taking beta-blockers and should be approached with caution.

Cevimeline is a new drug that also increases the production of saliva, and possibly of tears and other secretions. Like pilocarpine, cevimeline binds to cholinergic receptors, causing increased saliva secretion. The usual dosage is 30 mg orally three times a day. Its interactions and contraindications are similar to those of pilocarpine. Moreover, certain drugs that are also metabolized by the liver may increase cevimeline's activity: amiodarone, fluoxetine, paroxetine, quinidine, ritonavir, diltiazem, erythromycin, itraconazole, ketoconazole, and verapamil.

Abnormal contraction of the esophagus, known as esophageal dysmotility, can be treated with drugs that relax the smooth muscle of this part of the gastrointestinal tract. Nitroglycerine (0.3 to 0.6 mg, placed under the tongue) or longer-acting agents such as isosorbide dinitrate (10 to 30 mg orally before meals) and nifedipine (10 to 20 mg orally before meals) may be of benefit. Common side effects of nitrates are headache, light-headedness, and hypotension. Concurrent use of sildenafil is contraindicated because it lowers the blood pressure with nitrates. Calcium channel blockers such as nifedipine may also be used as treatment for esophageal dysmotility. They may cause flushing, leg swelling, dizziness, light-headedness, transient drop of the blood pressure, palpitations, nausea, and heartburn.

Gastroesophageal reflux may be treated initially with lifestyle modifications such as loss of weight, elevation of the head of the bed, eating smaller meals, avoidance of lying down within three hours of eating, and cessation of smoking and drinking if excessive. Mild acid reflux can be alleviated with administration of antacids. These act by forming a coat that protects the lining of the stomach and esophagus from the acids produced by the stomach; however, excessive use may result in diarrhea and increased levels of sodium, calcium, and magnesium in the blood.

Moreover, drugs that reduce acid production by the stomach are used for the treatment of acid reflux and esophagitis (inflammation of the esophagus caused by long-standing acid reflux). These drugs can be divided into two groups: H2 receptor antagonists, such as cimetidine, ranitidine, famotidine, and nizatidine, and proton pump inhibitors, such as omeprazole, lansoprazole, and pantoprazole. These drugs are generally preferred to antacids because they are more effective and have few side effects. However, some patients with Sjogren's already have reduced acid secretion in the stomach, due to the fact that the cells that produce acid have been destroyed by long-standing inflammation. This is known as chronic atrophic gastritis. In some patients it can result in pernicious anemia due to lack of a substance that is necessary for the absorption of vitamin B_{12}, which is important for the production of blood cells. Pernicious anemia is typically treated with intramuscular cyanocobalamin in a dose of 1,000 mcg (1 mg) every day for one week, followed by 1 mg every week for four weeks and then 1 mg every month for the remainder of the patient's life. Oral and nasal formulations are also available, but they require strict patient compliance. Monitoring of blood potassium level is necessary within the first few days of the initiation of treatment because a drop may occur due to increased utilization of potassium in the production of new blood cells.

Acute inflammation of the pancreas (acute pancreatitis) is a very rare complication of Sjogren's. Rarely, involvement of the pancreas may result in pancreatic enzyme deficiency, which is treated by oral administration of pancreatic enzymes, one to two capsules with each meal.

The Liver

Liver disease in primary Sjogren's syndrome is rare and mild, and most patients do not have any symptoms. Liver involvement can be suspected when there is elevation of the liver enzymes upon routine testing which is not attributed to medication. Primary biliary cirrhosis (PBC) is the most common liver disease associated with Sjogren's. It is characterized by an ongoing immunologic attack on the small bile ducts of the liver, which destroys their architecture and prevents the normal flow of bile acid from the liver into the intestine. This process eventually leads to scarring of the liver (cirrhosis) and liver failure. The presence of antimitochondrial antibodies (AMAs) in the blood is the most sensitive indicator of underlying liver pathology in primary Sjogren's syndrome patients. The management of PBC has two goals: treatment of the symptoms and complications that result from chronic cholestasis (obstruction of bile flow), and suppression of the underlying pathogenic process.

Itching of the skin (pruritus) is a common symptom in patients with PBC. It can often be controlled by nonspecific measures such as warm baths and emollients. If these measures fail, cholestyramine (4–16 g per day) and colestipol are usually effective in the treatment of moderate to severe pruritus. These drugs are nonabsorbable resins, which bind many substances in the gut lumen, including bile acids. However, they are relatively unpalatable, can induce constipation, and can interfere with the absorption of many drugs, including digoxin, warfarin, propanolol, and thiazide diuretics. Ursodeoxycholic acid (UDCA) is a naturally occurring bile acid that lowers bile acid levels and can help alleviate pruritus. Other modalities used for the same purpose are colchicine, methotrexate, and phototherapy.

Two forms of metabolic bone disease can occur in patients with primary biliary cirrhosis: osteoporosis and osteomalacia. The latter is now uncommon due to better dietary management and vitamin D supplementation. The diagnosis of osteoporosis is established by the demonstration of decreased bone mineral density. The administration of vitamin D is controversial, while calcium supplementation (to increase intake to at least 1,500 mg/day) is generally recommended because it is safe and avoids occult calcium deficiency in some patients. Administration of biphosphonates (e.g., alendronate) may also be effective in the treatment of osteoporosis. A high level of cholesterol in the blood (hypercholesterolemia) is a common feature of PBC and other forms of cholestatic liver disease. The available data suggest that patients with PBC are not at high risk for developing atherosclerosis. Thus administration of drugs to lower cholesterol levels remains controversial, and in some cases a low-fat diet may be adequate.

Patients with PBC may develop diarrhea and weight loss due to poor absorption of dietary fat (steatorrhea). This can be partially treated with restriction of fat intake. Medium-chain triglycerides (MCTs) may be added if caloric supplementation is required to maintain body weight. Each milliliter of MCT oil contains 7.5 calories, and most patients can tolerate a daily intake of 60 ml. This oil can be taken directly by the teaspoon or can be used as salad oil or in cooking.

Patients with PBC may malabsorb the fat-soluble vitamins A, D, E, and K. Deficiency of vitamin E is uncommon unless the disease is advanced. Many PBC patients do have a deficiency of vitamin A, but they are usually asymptomatic. They respond well with oral administration of 15,000 units per day, while parenteral supplementation may be necessary for those complaining of night blindness. If untreated, vitamin D deficiency may lead to osteomalacia. Vitamin K is important for blood clotting, but clinically important deficiency of vitamin K rarely occurs in PBC. Only patients with end-stage liver disease require vitamin K supplementation.

Approximately 20 percent of PBC patients have an underactive thyroid gland (hypothyroidism). The treatment of thyroid disorders is the same as in patients without Sjogren's syndrome. The most reliable test for diagnosis and follow-up of this disorder is the thyroid-stimulating hormone (TSH) blood level. Hypothyroidism is treated with thyroid hormone replacement at a dose that keeps TSH levels in the normal range.

Some PBC patients develop xanthomas, which are deposits of cholesterol in skin. Xanthelasmas, which are deposits of cholesterol in the skin folds around the eyes, are more common. These lesions develop in patients whose serum cholesterol exceeds 600 mg/dl (15.6 mmol) for more than three months. Planar xanthomas develop in the palms of the hands and in the soles of the feet and are painful. Because they can affect the patient's quality of life, planar xanthomas are usually treated. Treatment consists of large-volume plasmapheresis performed at one- to two-week intervals. Once the serum cholesterol level approaches normal, xanthomas will gradually resolve. This treatment is inconvenient, expensive, and indicated in only a small minority of patients with PBC. Most such patients undergo liver transplantation because of severe liver disease.

Portal hypertension (increased pressure in the portal vein, PHT) is a complication of cirrhosis and is treated with propanolol taken orally and sometimes by a surgical procedure in order to lower pressure in the portal vein.

There has been less success in treating the immune system's attack on the bile ducts in patients with PBC. A number of drugs have been shown to have little effect in slowing the disease. These include corticosteroids, penicillamine, cyclosporine, and azathioprine.

The drug ursodeoxycholic acid (13 to 15 mg per day) has been shown to delay the progression of PBC to end-stage liver disease. It improves patient survival and is well tolerated. Colchicine, a drug used for the treatment and prevention of gout, can also slow the rate of progression of PBC but does not stop it. It is contraindicated in serious kidney failure and in liver, heart, or blood disorders. Its main side effects are nausea, vomiting, diarrhea, and abdominal pain. When co-administered with vitamin B_{12} supplements, it reduces the absorption of the vitamin. Methotrexate, a drug that suppresses the immune system, may be helpful in PBC, but more trials are needed to establish its effectiveness.

In conclusion, suppression of the underlying disease in PBC remains still an unresolved problem, and some patients may eventually require liver transplantation. However, one must always keep in mind that PBC is most of the time mild or asymptomatic in Sjogren's patients; thus liver failure is really a very rare occurrence.

Other Systemic Manifestations and Therapies

NSAIDs can be taken by patients who suffer from mild to moderate joint pain (arthralgias). Their main side effects are indigestion, stomach pains, and water retention. Also, they can cause bleeding from stomach ulcers and therefore must not be given to people with a history of peptic ulcer. NSAIDs can affect the function of the liver and kidneys, and prolonged administration of these drugs should be avoided particularly in the elderly and those suffering from heart failure.

Antimalarial drugs (such as hydroxychloroquine at a dose of 200 to 400 mg daily) are used for mild systemic manifestations of Sjogren's such as inflammation of the joints, skin rashes, swollen glands, and fever; moreover, some investigators feel that they are disease-modifying agents. Hydroxychloroquine can take one to two years to have maximal effect, and there are controlled studies showing its efficacy. The most common side effects are nausea, vomiting, and (less usually) diarrhea. To lessen these problems one can slowly increase the daily dose of the drug or take it at bedtime. The advantage of using these drugs compared to NSAIDs is that they do not cause ulcer formation, bleeding from the stomach, or kidney failure. However, skin rashes as well as itching of the skin and mild allergic reactions may sometimes occur. Antimalarials, especially chloroquine, may rarely cause eye problems. Inability to focus, which resolves a few days after starting treatment, does not usually require discontinuation of the drug. Damage to the cells of the eye that perceive light (retinopathy) is a rare complication that occurs with high doses of the drug given for long periods of time; it can cause color blindness and blurred vision. If detected early, it is reversible with discontinuation of the drug. That is why a semiannual ophthalmologic examination is necessary for those patients taking antimalarials. Rarely, these drugs can affect the production of blood cells in the bone marrow. They should not be given in patients with deficiency of the enzyme G6PD, present in blood cells, because they can cause breaking of blood cells, known as hemolytic anemia. However, these drugs have been shown to be safe in pregnancy. No defects have been noted in newborns whose mothers were taking antimalarials while pregnant.

Propionic acid gels are sometimes given for the treatment of vaginal dryness. Dyspareunia (discomfort during sexual intercourse) is a common symptom among patients with Sjogren's syndrome. Use of vaginal moisturizing agents on a regular basis and lubricants before intercourse is recommended. A more effective therapy for postmenopausal women is vaginal estrogen therapy. This can help with vaginal dryness and stress incontinence (loss of urine) and can reduce the frequency of urinary tract infections.

Dryness of mouth, eyes, and vagina can lead to infections. Antibiotics may be necessary for bacterial parotitis and urinary tract infections. Candidiasis of the mouth and vagina is treated with antifungal agents (nystatin, clotrimazole) in the form of pills, oral gels, or vaginal suppositories.

Apart from drugs used for the alleviation of the symptoms of Sjogren's, other drugs, the so-called immunomodulators, may affect the progression of the disease and are usually used in patients with secondary Sjogren's syndrome. Azathioprine, cyclophosphamide, or mycophenolate are used together with steroids when severe but rare complications of Sjogren's occur, such as vasculitis, peripheral neuropathy, pericarditis, kidney involvement, and hemolytic anemia. As mentioned above, some investigators feel that antimalarials are immunomodulatory drugs as well.

Plasmapheresis may also be applied when a patient with Sjogren's syndrome suffers from peripheral neuropathy due to cryoglobulinemia. These patients suffer from numbness or burning sensations in their hands and feet or have muscle weakness. Immunosuppressive agents such as cyclophosphamide in combination with high-dose corticosteroids can also be used; dosage and method of administration are similar to those employed in glomerulonephritis.

In case of inflammation of the lining of the heart (pericarditis), the amount of fluid around the heart is usually mild to moderate and most

TABLE 16.1   DRUGS IN SJOGREN'S SYNDROME: SYMPTOMATIC TREATMENT

Generic name	Trade name	Indication
Bromhexine	*	Thinning secretions of the air tubes
Ambroxol	*	
Salbutamol (albuterol)	Ventolin	Bronchial dilation
Almitrine bismesylate	*	Interstitial lung disease
Nifedipine	Adalat	Pulmonary hypertension
Epoprostenol	Flolan	
Bosentan	Tracleer	
Amiloride	Midamor	Renal tubular acidosis
Triamterene	Dyrenium	
Spironolactone	Aldactone	
Pilocarpine	Salagen	Dry mouth and eyes
Cevimeline	Evoxac	
Nonsteroidal anti-inflammatory drugs, e.g., ibuprofen	Brufen	Arthralgias
Nitroglycerine		Esophageal dysmotility
Isosorbide dinitrate	Imdur	
Antacids, e.g., aluminium hydroxide gel	Maalox Aludrox	Acid reflux and esophagitis
Cimetidine	Tagamet	
Ranitidine	Zantac	
Nizatidine	Axid	
Omeprazole	Prilosec	
Lansoprazole	Prevacid	
Pancreatic enzymes	Cotazym	Pancreatic enzyme deficiency
Cyanocobalamin	Dicopac	Pernicious anemia
Cholestyramine	Questran	Pruritus in primary biliary cirrhosis (PBC)
Colestipol	Colestid	
Alendronate	Fosamax	Osteoporosis in PBC
Vitamin D		
Medium-chain triglycerides	Tazorac	Maintaining body weight in PBC

continued

Generic name	Trade name	Indication
Vitamin A		Vitamin malabsorption in PBC
Vitamin K	Aqua-Mephyton	Rarely in end-stage liver disease
Ursodeoxycholic acid	Ursofalk	Inhibition of progression of PBC
Levothyroxine		Hypothyroidism
Vaginal estrogen therapy		Vaginal dryness
Antibiotics, e.g., tetracycline, amoxycillin		Bacterial infection of the parotid glands and urinary tract infections
Antifungal agents, e.g., nystatin, clotrimazole	Mycostatin, Mycelex	Fungal infection of the mouth and vagina

*Not available in the United States

TABLE 16.2 DRUGS IN SJOGREN'S SYNDROME: IMMUNOMODULATORY EFFECT

Generic name	Trade name	Indication
Corticosteroids, e.g., prednisone, methylprednisolone	Deltasone Medrol	Interstitial lung disease (ILD), glomerulonephritis, PBC, pleuritis, pericarditis
Azathioprine	Imuran	ILD, PBC, pericarditis
Cyclophosphamide	Cytoxan	ILD, glomerulonephritis, peripheral neuropathy, vasculitis, hemolytic anemia, cryoglobulinemia
Cyclosporine	Sandimmune Neoral	ILD, PBC
Mycophenolate mofetil	Cellcept	Glomerulonephritis
Methotrexate	Folex, Nexate	PBC
Antimalarials, e.g., hydroxychloroquine	Plaquenil	Rash, arthralgias

of the time subsides with the use of drugs. Oral steroids at a dose of 1 mg/kg are used together with a steroid-sparing drug such as azathioprine. In this way tapering of corticosteroids becomes easier thereafter.

Tables 16.1 and 16.2 summarize some of the agents reviewed in this chapter.

Jeanne L. Melvin, MS, OTR/L, FAOTA

17 Taming Sjogren's: Fighting Fatigue, Lifestyle Factors, and Nondrug Management

ONCE A PERSON DEVELOPS a serious illness or condition that cannot be cured with medication or surgery, it is extremely helpful to approach healing from a very broad, holistic perspective that will strengthen overall health and the immune system in addition to treating or reducing the specific symptoms. This process is called self-management.

The four cornerstones of optimal health are restorative sleep, healthy nutrition, exercise that promotes cardiovascular fitness, and positive mood. Improving health in these areas constitutes a wellness approach to treating autoimmune disorders such as Sjogren's syndrome, rheumatoid arthritis, lupus, and noninflammatory conditions including fibromyalgia. This chapter focuses on how patients can use these behaviors to improve overall health.

Fatigue

Fatigue is one of the most common symptoms for which people with Sjogren's syndrome and other rheumatic diseases request help. My patients tell me, "I could cope with the pain and other symptoms if I just weren't so tired. It is fatigue that gets me down." Fatigue can be affected by sleep, level of inflammation, level of physical fitness, stress, depression, and nutrition. Table 17.1 illustrates some common fatigue patterns.

TABLE 17.1   CAUSES OF FATIGUE AND COMMON PATTERNS OF FATIGUE

- **Deconditioning**—fatigue following minimal level of any physical activity
- **Depression**—fatigue all the time, no matter how much sleep; often worst in the morning; person may sleep excessively (10 or more hours)
- **Fibromyalgia syndrome (FMS)**—wake up feeling tired, exhausted, or unrefreshed; best energy in the afternoon
- **Osteoarthritis (OA)**—fatigue at end of day, early evening, or after physical activity
- **Rheumatoid arthritis (RA)**—fatigue in early afternoon, refreshed by nap; systemic fatigue resulting from disease flare, usually lasts all day and is not resolved with a nap
- **Systemic lupus erythematosus (SLE)**—fatigue, exhaustion, not resolved with sleep; lessens with control of disease

---

Fatigue Management Training

Prior to the mid-1980s, the primary rehabilitation approach to treating fatigue associated with rheumatic diseases was energy conservation training. It simply taught people how to conserve their limited energy resources. Then research on exercise and arthritis demonstrated that people with rheumatoid arthritis, osteoarthritis, lupus, and fibromyalgia could improve their fitness level and functional ability through proper exercise. Now fatigue management training for people with rheumatic diseases includes fitness exercise training in addition to education of effective use of time and energy. Time management, planning, pacing, and prioritizing are actually more helpful than just energy conservation for people with Sjogren's syndrome. Also, many over-the-counter and prescription medications can cause fatigue or disturb sleep. Check with your physician or pharmacist, for there are sometimes alternatives. In addition to exercise, healthy sleep and good nutrition are critical to managing fatigue.

To start a fatigue management program, patients should start on a healthy diet, get involved with an aerobic fitness exercise program (see Table 17.2), and do everything possible to eliminate factors that impair sleep. The program should be undertaken for at least 12 weeks; if no improvement is evident after that time, the doctor should be consulted about a referral to a sleep specialist or rehabilitation program that does fatigue management training.

TABLE 17.2	TECHNIQUES FOR THE MANAGEMENT OF FATIGUE

Exercise
Sleep
Time management, pacing, prioritizing
Energy conservation
Healthy nutrition
Evaluation of medications that can cause fatigue

Sleep and Fatigue

Most people with autoimmune disorders have been told that fatigue is part of the disorder, so they just assume that the illness is the source of their fatigue and they try to accept it. If they have obvious insomnia, they may see it as a cause of their fatigue. But if they sleep through the night and wake tired, they think the illness is causing the fatigue. But often the real problem is that these people have poor-quality sleep that is not deep enough and therefore is nonrestorative. Sleep starts with light, stage 1 sleep and progresses to deep, stage 4 sleep followed by a phase called rapid eye movement (REM) sleep. This cycle takes about 90 minutes and then repeats. There are about six cycles in an eight-hour period. Stage 4 sleep is called restorative sleep because although the body is very quiet, the brain turns into a chemical factory, producing essential neurochemicals such as serotonin, growth hormone, and cortisol, among many others. People can sleep soundly in stage 3 sleep, but if they don't get enough of stage 4 sleep, they can wake up tired, irritable, and achy. When a person's mood is irritable, the entire body is hypersensitive or irritable.

People can tell that they have had enough stage 4 sleep if they wake up feeling mentally rested and restored. How rested someone feels is more important than how many hours are slept or how many awakenings occur during the night. So here are some options to consider.

Possibility #1: *The patient sleeps an ideal number of hours most nights and wakes feeling mentally rested five out of seven mornings without sleeping pills, antihistamines, or alcohol but has fatigue during the day.* In this case, the patient probably has good-quality sleep; poor sleep is not the source of the fatigue. Other factors such as pain, deconditioning, stress, depression, nutritional factors, or simply overdoing and not pacing could be contributing to the fatigue, in addition to systemic inflammation from the autoimmune disorder itself.

Possibility #2: *The patient sleeps an ideal number of hours without using sleeping pills but wakes feeling tired or exhausted.* In this case, the patient may have nonrestorative sleep. Improving the quality of sleep would likely reduce fatigue.

The most common factors that reduce quality of sleep and are easy to fix are (1) caffeine (which can stay in the system for 20 hours), (2) sleeping with the TV or a light on, (3) having windows that let light in at night or in the early morning, as seeing white light (even when using the bathroom) stops the secretion of sleep hormone (melatonin), (4) doing exercise too close to bedtime, (5) doing work activities in the hour before bed (not allowing enough time to wind down), (6) eating late, heavy meals, (7) drinking alcohol after dinner (alcohol causes fragmented sleep at night), (8) and mattresses that are too firm or sagging.

Factors that are more difficult to fix are (1) smoking (nicotine disturbs sleep), (2) pets on the bed, (3) use of antidepressant medications such as selective serotonin reuptake inhibitors, (4) children that need attending, (5) partners who snore, (6) noise from neighbors, (7) arguing or having stressful phone calls right before bed, (8) bladder disorders, and (9) use of corticosteroid medications for asthma or autoimmune disorders. For some people, not getting regular exercise reduces sleep quality. Taking a warm bath in the evening can be helpful, but a hot bath too close to sleep time can increase core temperature and make it difficult to cool down sufficiently to fall asleep easily. The same results can occur with exercise, so vigorous exercise should be done at least three hours before bedtime. A relaxing walk in the evening often helps people relax and sleep better, and gentle stretching before bed can help reduce morning stiffness in patients with arthritis. Medications that cause insomnia should be taken as early in the day as possible. If there is any suspicion that medications or pain are disturbing sleep, talk to the doctor, and see the section on pain below.

Having healthy sleep means being able to go to sleep when desired, returning to sleep easily after awakening, sleeping as long as desired, and waking up feeling mentally rested. This is possible without taking medication or alcohol for sleep. Patients may not want to face the challenges of the day and may not be energetic, but they feel rested, as if they have had enough sleep. And this feeling lasts longer than a few minutes. Ideally, it lasts through the whole morning.

If a patient has daytime fatigue and snores or has a sense of stopping breathing or having difficulty breathing at night, the doctor should be consulted. Sleep apnea (a type of abnormal breathing during sleep) is a disorder that can cause these symptoms, and it is treatable with an oxygen device, surgery, or a dental appliance.

White light from a TV, night-light, or the moon can disturb sleep. It is darkness that triggers the secretion of melatonin, the sleep hormone. An inexpensive way to test whether moonlight is a problem is to use a nighttime eye shade (a soft satin one with an extra piece to block light from the sides of your nose is better than a stiff eyeshade). The ones distributed on airlines work well. Red light does not disturb sleep in the way white light does.

Sleep Medications

The key to using sleep for maintaining or restoring health is to be able to sleep deeply and wake feeling rested without drugs. When this occurs, the body and the brain are in balance, and the biochemical "switch" in the brain that allows a person to go from wakefulness to sleep is working. Taking drugs at night may help somewhat to increase sleep, but they do not fix a switch that is not working. They bypass the natural sleep process and induce sleep through an artificial or alternative pathway, so the body continues out of balance, and any health problems to which this contributes remain. Medications can sometimes serve as a stepping-stone to correcting a problem, but they should not be the destination. (There are some exceptions to this rule, such as medications for severe anxiety disorders and other mental illness.) The way to "fix the switch" is by changing the physiology of the brain. This can be done through exercise, relaxation training, nutrition, sleep, and even changing one's attitude toward something. For example, say on a particular Saturday a patient gets a lot of enjoyable exercise and that night sleeps great, far better than usual. This is because the exercise changed the physiology of the brain and improved the working of the biochemical switches necessary for deep sleep. Pills cannot do this because they create sleep through an artificial pathway. Drug-induced sleep is not the same as or as good as natural sleep; all sleep specialists are in agreement on this issue. Some sleeping pills may also make dry eye and dry mouth worse.

It has only been during the last 20 years that science has begun to uncover new and surprising facts about the purposes of sleep. A few years ago it was thought that the main purpose of sleep was simply to give the body a rest. But now we know that although the body seems quiet during deep sleep, the chemistry lab of the brain is in high gear, replenishing the neurochemicals that control all the body's functions, including mood, heartbeat, and digestion. And the greatest amount of cellular repair in the body occurs during deep sleep. This makes deep sleep one of the most essential elements in maintaining general health, both mental and physical.

Nutrition

Daily fatigue, chronic pain, poor sleep, or fibromyalgia are signs that the body's chemistry is out of balance. The good news is that the body is always trying to bring its chemistry back into balance. Good nutrition and vitamins can help the body win this battle. Good nutrition can influence mood, energy level, thinking ability, and sleep. It is not simply a matter of eating a certain food or taking a certain vitamin and having the Sjogren's syndrome go away or the fibromyalgia and lupus disappear. It is a matter of eating to increase health and stamina and to improve the chemistry in the body, including the brain. Any pattern of foods or supplementation that reduces symptoms is probably improving body chemistry.

People with fatigue problems or fibromyalgia often report that they have developed increased sensitivity to everything, especially medications and drugs such as caffeine and alcohol. Many patients stop drinking alcoholic beverages because alcohol makes them feel awful. Some people report a new sensitivity to certain foods, such as sugar, other sweeteners, chocolate, and red meat. They feel worse after eating these foods. It can be very helpful to pay attention to responses to foods and eliminate any that increase symptoms. If it seems that several foods may be problematic but it is not clear which ones, it is helpful to work with a nutritionist, who can design an elimination or cleansing diet that lasts for two weeks, followed by a process of reintroducing foods to the diet one at a time so that the response to each can be evaluated. Look at how foods affect pain, fatigue, sleep, alertness, energy, and mood. A word of caution: if a certain food makes one or more symptoms worse, it does not mean that the patient is allergic to that food. He or she may just be sensitive to or intolerant of it. Stress, poor sleep, depression, and fibromyalgia can make the system hypersensitive to the substance, similar to the way it may be hypersensitive to touch, sound, or other irritants. As health improves, tolerance to these foods is likely to improve.

Here are some of the basic nutritional guidelines to reduce the symptoms of fatigue, irritability, and hypersensitivity and help the body achieve optimal health:

Nutrition and Fatigue

Tiredness can exacerbate depression, anxiety, or irritableness and lower motivation for participating in activities or exercise. Most nutritionists agree that eating a healthy diet (one low in fats, sugar, and additives but with adequate protein and high in complex carbohydrates from vegetables, whole grains, and fruits) helps improve energy, mood, and motivation, allowing a person to participate in more physical activities, which in turn reduces stress and improves sleep. If a person is feeling energetic, he or she is more likely to exercise during the day. Eating a high-protein, low-fat breakfast and lunch can improve energy and stamina for the day. It can also help in weight loss by increasing energy and metabolism so that calories burn off faster. (See Table 17.3 defining food categories.)

The type of meal that maximizes alertness and ability to respond quickly is a high-protein (12 or more grams), low-fat (20 percent of calories from fat) meal. Studies have shown that eating this type of meal at breakfast and lunch can improve mental alertness by increasing levels of the neurochemicals dopamine and noradrenaline, which are made from the amino acid tyrosine.

Food can influence sleep in several ways. In the evening and before bed certain foods can interfere with sleep, and others can facilitate sleep.

Foods That Interfere with Sleep

When taken too close to bedtime, highly acidic foods, such as tomatoes, oranges, grapefruit, and citrus juices, can disrupt sleep. Acidic foods are stimulants, which is why they are associated with breakfast and make a great natural pick-me-up in the late afternoon. Herbal teas

---

TABLE 17.3   FOOD CATEGORIES

Complex Carbohydrates

Whole grains: rice, corn, oatmeal, wheat
Vegetables
Beans (legumes), fresh and dried
Fruits, including avocado
Starches: potatoes, rice, breads, pasta

Simple Carbohydrates

Sweets: candy, sodas, cookies, cake, pie, pastry
Sugar, syrup, honey

Good Sources of Protein

Animal products: meat, chicken, fish
Eggs
Dairy: milk, yogurt, cottage cheese
Soy beans, tofu, and vegetarian "meats" (tofu dogs, bacon, etc.)
Fruit juice smoothies made with protein powder, milk, or yogurt

High-Fat Foods

Oils, butter, margarine, mayonnaise, salad dressing
Fried foods: potato chips, corn chips, doughnuts, french fries
Fatty meats: bacon, sausage, salami, bologna, hot dogs
Olives
Nuts
Ice cream

---

that contain citrus can also interfere with sleep. Multivitamins and B-complex vitamins, both of which increase energy, and vitamin C supplements, which are acidic, can all interfere with sleep. They should be taken with breakfast or lunch to enhance energy. Cayenne pepper, horseradish, and other hot spices are also "uppers" that can interfere with sleep. People with Sjogren's syndrome generally avoid these substances because they are irritating and drying.

Optimal hydration is critical to good health and hardiness. Dehydration can interfere with sleep. (On the other hand, too much liquid before bed can interrupt sleep by necessitating trips to the bathroom.) Seven to eight glasses of water or noncaffeinated drinks are recommended a day (caffeine is a diuretic). One of the first signs of dehydration is fatigue. Patients who are tired should take account of how much water they have had and should drink a glass of water to see if it increases energy and alertness.

Eating foods that are hard to digest, such as raw apples, nuts, popcorn, raw vegetables, or spicy foods, right before bed can interfere with sleep. Dieting and going to bed hungry can also interfere with sleep.

Alcohol is a commonly used sleep aid, but it is not a good one. It has a calming, sleep-inducing effect, but it results in fragmented sleep and can cause rebound insomnia after just a few hours of sleep. Also, alcohol is a diuretic and encourages dehydration, and it increases the symptoms of restless-leg syndrome and can simply make people more restless in bed. It is better to have wine or another alcoholic drink with an early dinner and have nonalcoholic, decaffeinated drinks between dinner and sleep. Also, optimal hydration helps reduce the negative effects of alcohol on your body.

Caffeine requires special consideration. It is a long-acting drug that can profoundly interfere with sound sleep. Some people are very aware that caffeine makes them feel jittery or irritates their stomach, aggravates irritable bowel syndrome, or interferes with their sleep. They gladly give it up to feel better. For others, especially people addicted to caffeine or those who used to drink it before going to bed at night, the connection between caffeine and poor sleep seems remote and not applicable to them. But once a sleep disorder has developed, the system becomes hypersensitive, and the body's response to caffeine (or nicotine or alcohol) can change. When a patient has difficulty sleeping or wakes up tired in the morning, the best thing to do is to avoid all caffeine, including that contained in coffee, tea, sodas, chocolate, cocoa, and over-the-counter medications such as Excedrin. Patients who continue to have problems sleeping should wean themselves from all caffeine. People who are addicted to caffeine need to reduce consumption gradually to avoid withdrawal headaches. Decaffeinated coffee contains between 3 and 10 percent of the caffeine of regular coffee, depending on the brand and brew method (Sanka has the lowest amount at 1 percent). Both regular and decaffeinated coffees are very acidic drinks. Acid is an irritant to the digestive tract and a stimulant to muscles, increasing tightness. (Also, caffeine contributes to calcium loss in the bones, which is of concern to women at risk for osteoporosis.)

Foods That Can Help Sleep

Foods that increase serotonin and muscle relaxation may promote sleep. A carbohydrate snack such as cookies low in sugar, graham crackers, saltines, bread, or rice cakes with a little jam can increase serotonin in the brain. Eating a protein snack tends to increase energy and interfere with the production of serotonin. Milk, however, even though it supplies protein, is effective as a bedtime snack. Milk may help people relax because it is high in calcium, which reduces acidity in the body and is thought to be calming. It is also high in magnesium, which can reduce muscle tension and blood pressure.

Chocoholics with desperate cravings in the evening should try white chocolate, which contains no caffeine.

Smoking

Although nicotine is not a nutritional substance, it can alter nutrition and body chemistry. Nicotine constricts blood flow in the small capillaries, reducing circulation in the hands, feet, face, and muscles. It is a poison to the body and creates an unhealthy chemical imbalance. And it is a stimulant that interferes with sleep.

Very tense patients who smoke to relax, or who smoke more when depressed or worried, should talk to a physician about the possibility of nondrying antidepressant medications to encourage relaxation while withdrawing from nicotine.

Stress Management

I have met many people with illness who refuse to participate in stress-management classes because they know what is causing their stress—for example, their marriage, children, job, or boss—and know they cannot get rid of these problems. But the goal of stress management is not to get rid of all stress, which is impossible, but instead to learn how to handle stress so that it does not affect the body physically in the form of headaches, insomnia, tight muscles, rashes, high blood pressure, nervousness (anxiety), depression, and so on. In other words, if stress is having a physical effect, it is not being handled well. Stress can magnify or compound the symptoms of Sjogren's syndrome, fibromyalgia, rheumatoid arthritis, or lupus.

Stress management training can take many forms, but classes and individual therapy generally include the following:

1 Guidance in how to identify big and small stresses

2 Education on how stress affects the body and health

3 Identifying how stress is handled, the types of stress that are handled well, and the types that result in physical symptoms

4 Techniques to manage anger or communicate effectively (assertiveness training)

5 New ways to think about stressful events so that they cause less reaction (cognitive-behavioral therapy, which includes techniques to help stop the mind from worrying and obsessing about problems or stopping the mind from racing)

6 Time management skills, including prioritizing activities

7 Relaxation methods to regain control over your body and relax the muscles at will

Hydration Management

This topic covers the full array of self-management strategies to improve systemic hydration, increase humidity in the environment, and maximize moisture for eyes, mouth, and skin. The most obvious way to improve systemic hydration is to drink enough liquids. Most people with Sjogren's or dry skin in general find it helpful to use a humidifier in the home and especially in the bedroom at night. These need regular cleaning, so the best model is one that is easy to clean.

The brain is very reactive to the environmental atmosphere. That is why we can become irritable in rooms that are too warm or during periods of dry, hot winds. Air rich in negatively charged ions may have a refreshing and calming effect on us and increase brain serotonin. The greatest amount of negative ions are at the base of a waterfall, which is one reason they have such a calming effect on people. At night, the best environment for sleeping is with the air cool and the blankets warm. Of course, people with Raynaud's phenomenon need a temperature that works best for their circulation. The early morning, when there is dew on the ground, and the early evening, after it cools down, are also atmospheres with greater negative ions, so these are ideal times to take a relaxing or invigorating walk.

Specific techniques for enhancing moisture for the eyes, skin, and mouth are covered in Appendix 3.

Pain Management

Poor sleep or nonrestorative sleep, depression, anxiety, lack of exercise, and unhealthy nutrition can all magnify the pain signals. This process is called pain amplification.

In health care, pain management refers to a program that teaches patients how to gain control over pain by reducing factors that magnify or aggravate pain. Pain management programs include:

1 Techniques for reducing anxiety, stress, and depression

2 Learning to let go of the fear of a flare of pain or progression of pain by learning self-management of symptoms

3 Learning to reduce pain and suffering by understanding the response to symptoms, setting goals, and having methods for determining progress so that the focus can be on progress instead of problems

4 Counseling or psychotherapy to help cope with losses related to illness and developing plans to maximize the possibility of a productive and satisfying life even though not all the pain may be gone

Rehabilitation Professionals and Services

Physical Therapy

Ideally, people should participate in a community fitness program on a regular basis. If this is difficult, a physical therapist can help patients design a fitness program and show them how to gradually increase exercise with the goal of participating in a community program.

Physical therapy can alleviate a localized physical problem contributing to pain, such as trigger points or a specific tight muscle. When the main problem is generalized stiffness and discomfort, as in fibromyalgia, a total-body stretching and toning exercise program is the most effective.

For neck and back stiffness, physical therapists can apply specific manual techniques to release tight muscles. Physical therapists can teach deep breathing, relaxation, and self-massage techniques. They can explain how to use devices that allow the application of focal pressure to release trigger points at home.

Occupational Therapy

Occupational therapists are concerned with patients' ability to do activities that occupy their time, mind, and hands—that is, the functional activities that occupy the day. This may include a vocation, but it is not limited to work activities. Occupational therapists are trained in the fields of both physical rehabilitation and psychiatry. They can offer a wide range of services that can help both physically and emotionally.

Occupational therapists can help patients evaluate their daily routine, to see whether their method for carrying out activities is helping or hindering healing. In many pain programs, occupational therapists teach stress management, fatigue management, sleep hygiene, assertiveness training, values clarification, joint protection techniques, time management, and planning and pacing skills, all techniques that can help reduce pain, stress, anxiety, and fatigue. If job or home activities are contributing to an increase in neck, back, or arm pain, an occupational therapist can evaluate workstation, methods, and postural stress and make specific recommendations for reducing the strain on the body. The majority of hand therapists are occupational therapists, and they can provide specific therapy, custom splints, and exercises for hand, elbow, and shoulder pain. The overall goal of occupational therapy is to improve the ability to carry out daily activities and to reduce disability.

Psychotherapy

A psychotherapist is a health professional who uses a variety of psychological therapy techniques to help patients understand the issues that may be contributing to depression, anxiety, and poor sleep. They can help patients understand and manage stress and pain better. A psychotherapist may be a psychiatrist, psychologist, social worker, or counselor.

Seeing a psychotherapist does not mean the symptoms are all in the patient's head; rather, it helps the patient understand that emotions and stress can affect level of pain or symptoms, and helps the patient take advantage of the latest techniques and research in psychology to help reduce symptoms. See Chapter 18 for further discussion.

Biofeedback

Biofeedback is a treatment that allows patients to see on a computer screen or machine how tense the muscles are. This feedback allows patients to learn effective techniques for reducing muscle tension or emotional distress. With this method, it is also possible to teach patients how to raise their body temperature, which can be helpful for managing Raynaud's phenomenon. Biofeedback can also be beneficial for management of headaches, jaw pain (temporomandibular joint syndrome), teeth grinding, and high blood pressure. It is administered by health professionals who are certified biofeedback technicians, or by other professionals such as occupational or physical therapists and psychologists who are certified to do so.

Joan E. Broderick, PhD

Evelyn J. Bromet, PhD

18 Conquering Sjogren's

IN THIS CHAPTER, we discuss anger, depression, fatigue, and chronic pain, four critical issues that Sjogren's patients often face on a daily basis. We then consider strategies for managing these challenges.

Jane's Story

Jane was a family court attorney who was enjoying the last few years of her law practice. The youngest of her three children was a sophomore in high school, enabling Jane to devote herself more fully to her work. For the past 20 years, she had successfully juggled raising young children and working part time representing abused and neglected children in family court proceedings. She was passionate about her work and was delighted with the new opportunities to sit on committees and conduct professional workshops to promote improved care for these vulnerable children. Despite working more hours professionally, Jane remembers commenting to her husband that she was feeling less stressed in her life than she had been 10 years earlier, when she was juggling more responsibilities at home and with the children. The increased freedom to throw herself fully into her work was exhilarating. At the same time, menopause was around the corner, and Jane was beginning to notice the small physical changes that accompany it: dry and sagging skin, less vaginal lubrication, less energy, some mood swings, and of course changes in her cycle. But, as Jane tells the story, she was taking this in stride, as she had most of the minor physical ailments that had come and gone through her life. These little annoyances were trivial compared with the suffering she had observed in her sister, who had been struggling for the past eight years with lupus, and in her aunt, who had been crippled by rheumatoid arthritis. However, as time progressed, even though she was through menopause, the symptoms were not lessening. Rather, they were getting worse. Now her eyes were gritty and dry, she was awakening repeatedly during the night with a parched mouth, and for the first time she was experiencing chronic heartburn and frequent constipation. Worst of all was the overwhelming fatigue that made getting through her day feel like she was trying to scale Mt. Everest. Jane was bewildered and self-critical. Everyone says that getting old is hard, but why was she handling it so poorly? She loved her job, her children were becoming competent young adults, and she and her husband still enjoyed each other's company. It was a visit to her dentist for a toothache that began the journey to a diagnosis. Dr. Jacobs, her dentist, remarked that she was developing decay at the gum line and on the incisal edges of her front teeth. He recommended that Jane see her primary care doctor for a full checkup. Blood tests revealed that Jane's rheumatoid factor and ANA were elevated. The journey continued with a consultation with a rheumatologist, who eventually made the diagnosis of Sjogren's syndrome. At first Jane was relieved to finally have a medical explanation for why she had been feeling so awful. Then the deeper implications began to sink in. Sjogren's is a chronic illness with few treatment options available. There was going to be little her doctor could do to reduce her symptoms of dryness or fatigue. This was a life sentence! She couldn't fathom what she had done to deserve this. It was so unfair. Finally at the point in her life when she had the opportunity to focus on her own interests and enjoy life with fewer responsibilities, it was being stolen away from her. Jane began to struggle with anger and depression.

Anger

Anger is an inevitable reaction to having a chronic illness. Our parents and teachers told us that life isn't fair, but developing a chronic disease such as Sjogren's syndrome was not what anyone bargained for. Most of us believe that if we work hard and conduct ourselves with reasonable moral integrity, then we will enjoy the fruits and blessings that come with that. The plaintive "Why me?" reverberates over and over in the mind of the newly diagnosed patient. "What did I do to deserve this?" is the question that prompts the answer "Nothing" and generates the anger. We can all think of people who abused their bodies for years through poor nutrition, smoking, substance abuse, or no exercise but whose health seems unaffected by these behaviors.

Human nature drives us to search for causal explanations for important events in our lives. We need to make sense of how personal choices and external events determine our subsequent experience. We draw lessons from these explanations such that we feel that we can exert a reasonable amount of control over what happens in our life. Most of us share the general view that when bad things happen to people, they probably contributed to it one way or the other. They lived in the wrong neighborhood, didn't work hard enough, lacked self-control, were self-indulgent, or didn't have sufficient moral character. We are constantly bombarded by news reports about how our choices and our environment determine our health. Headlines scream at us that being overweight leads to diabetes, heart disease, and certain types of cancer. Smoking leads to cancer, heart disease, stroke, and emphysema. Lack of exercise contributes to high cholesterol, fatigue, and diminished conditioning that makes daily tasks more difficult to complete as we age. Insufficient calcium results in accelerated bone loss with the consequence of increased risk of bone fractures, most importantly hip fractures, and osteoporosis. Especially in the United States, we are avid consumers of health news in our effort to try to take control of our destiny.

Given this context, it is not surprising that individuals diagnosed with Sjogren's syndrome, like many patients with chronic illness, inflict intense examination on themselves to uncover the root causes of their illness: "What did I do wrong? How did I bring this on myself? What should I have done differently to prevent this illness? How are women who didn't get this illness different from me?" When the answers are not satisfying, anger follows. "I've lived my life as well as anyone else. There is no good reason for me to have gotten Sjogren's. I have been betrayed!" This sense of betrayal can profoundly challenge our spiritual beliefs as well as our view of our bodies.

For most of us as children, our bodies worked like an exquisite Swiss watch. It ran almost perfectly, with just an occasional cold or childhood illness. A scraped knee, a broken arm, or a pulled muscle were the only times we paid any attention to our body. During puberty our body began to behave in surprising ways, but we easily assimilated these changes into our emerging self-identity. For the healthy individual, body and self are one and the same; there is no dichotomy or divergence. This is not so for the patient struggling with an illness. What emerges is an internal splitting: there is "me," and separate from that is "my body," which is behaving poorly. The "me" feels profoundly betrayed by "my body." Anger, disappointment, and frustration with "my body" are all anger directed at the self. We experience ourselves as defective. We demand that our body get its act together, because we will not tolerate this poor performance. When this does not happen, we are outraged.

The most virulent anger is that directed toward the self, but it is not limited to that. Many patients with Sjogren's syndrome and other chronic illness gradually develop pervasive anger at the health care establishment and particularly past and present health care providers. "Why did it take so long for me to be diagnosed?" "I knew it wasn't all in my head; how dare they keep telling me that I was just depressed or stressed with my teenage children." "I waited three months for this visit with the specialist (not to mention the hour and a half in his crowded waiting room) and then spent no more than 10 minutes with the doctor, who wouldn't take the time to answer all of my questions and didn't have any useful recommendations other than to do my best to live with it. I got more answers from a Web site!" "I am tired of being made to feel like a psychologically dysfunctional malcontent when I go to doctors trying to figure out what my symptoms are about and what I can do about them. 'It's just your Sjogren's, stop worrying about it' makes me feel that I am wasting the doctor's time and that I am coping poorly." The ride home from the office is dominated by tearful anger at the doctor, resurgence of anger at "my body," and now the added anger at "the self" for coping so poorly.

Sadness and Depression

It is not surprising that many patients with a chronic medical illness also experience depression. For many Sjogren's patients, the pain, fatigue, and other symptoms that come with the disease exhaust their emotional resources, and depression sets in. Moreover, diminished performance in meaningful life tasks, be it care of one's home, child care, employment, or hobbies, creates a sense of deep loss and disappointment. Chronic illnesses such as Sjogren's almost always require that the patient engage in a process of redefining the self from the pre-illness state to the current illness state. From the patient's point of view, this new self is inadequate because in so many areas it is less capable than the former, healthy self. A sense of loss is pervasive. Not only is the patient suffering from the physical symptoms of the disease, but she is also suffering from the loss of important positive experiences at home, on the job, with friends, and with hobbies that used to provide much enjoyment and personal fulfillment. In some cases the losses can be severe, through partial or full disability for employment and through separation, divorce, or other ended relationships.

When depression becomes persistent and impairing, it is a medical illness, not a moral failing, as many people imply. Research has discovered that when a person develops clinical depression, many changes occur throughout the body. Sleep is affected through disrupted patterns in brain wave activity, frequent nighttime awakenings associated with difficulty returning to sleep, and a feeling of exhaustion even after a full night of rest. Digestion becomes sluggish, appetite can increase or decrease substantially, and weight gain or weight loss is common. Speech and movement can become noticeably slower. The neurochemical and hormonal balances are altered, along with the functioning of the immune system. These physiological changes are accompanied by the well-known psychological symptoms of depression. Patients experience sadness, guilt, hopelessness, a sense of personal failure, and pessimism about the future. Pleasure from enjoyable activities, including sex, is markedly less. Toxic thoughts predominate, with a sense of worthlessness and shame that can progress to the belief that one would be better off dead, if for no better reason than to end the suffering. Family and coworkers will take note of many of these symptoms but will probably be most disturbed by the chronic irritability. When a patient has five or more such symptoms lasting at least two weeks, we determine that the person is suffering from a clinical depression rather than the garden-variety fluctuations in mood that we all experience in times of stress. Whereas most of us will rapidly get over these transient mood disturbances and are usually able to distract ourselves or otherwise help make ourselves feel better, a patient with clinical depression can do neither. Just as we can't will ourselves to lower our cholesterol, increase our insulin, or mend our damaged heart valve, neither can depressed patients will themselves to snap out of their depression, no matter how hard they may try. For a doctor, a family member, or the patient herself to suggest that is to add insult to injury.

Studies report that at any given time approximately 6–8 percent of people in the United States suffer from depression. In primary care patients, however, the rate is closer to 30–50 percent. Sjogren's patients are not immune from this. Indeed, a recent survey of the membership of the Sjogren's Syndrome Foundation (SSF) found that 29 percent reported depression as one of their most troubling problems.

Sjogren's presents a unique challenge to the treatment of depression by virtue of its primary symptom, dryness. Antidepressant medication is the most common tool for treating depression. Although medication can take several weeks to achieve its therapeutic effect, and patient and physician may need to tinker with more than one medication, research finds that 80 percent of depressed patients will experience a significant improvement in their depression with antidepressant therapy. However, many antidepressant medications have anticholinergic effects that result in dry mouth and constipation. These side effects are mild and generally well tolerated by many patients, but for the Sjogren's patient, they are often intolerable, making such patients poor candidates for this form of drug treatment. Many complementary medicines also have side effects. For example, St. John's wort (*Hypericum perforatum*) can increase photosensitivity and cause dry mouth as well. Depending on the situation, individual or group counseling may be a more desirable form of treatment.

Fatigue

Fatigue is another very distressing symptom associated with Sjogren's. Fatigue was the third most common symptom, after dry eye and dry mouth, reported in the SSF 1998 survey, with 77 percent of members listing it as one of their most troubling symptoms. The fatigue that patients with chronic illness describe is not the same as the tiredness that people without such an illness feel after staying up too late or putting in a long day of yard work. It goes much deeper, as though most of our life force has been drained away. It can feel like we have a three-ton gorilla on our back, so just moving about and doing the simplest tasks require all the energy we can muster. Waking up in the morning and already feeling totally exhausted can be very discouraging.

A couple of points are worth noting. First, we need to become good observers of the patterns that are associated with fluctuations in our levels of fatigue, either increasing or decreasing. A very typical pattern is seen in the patient who has been having a stretch of fatigue and then has a couple of days of more energy. Like a kid at a carnival, the patient jumps for joy and runs around doing all kinds of things. This overdoing can often result in a big crash with severe fatigue. Pacing is a strategy that is very helpful at avoiding this seesaw effect. It involves maintaining a level of activity that is punctuated with quieter, restful times regardless of how much energy we seem to have at the moment. It functions to keep us from drifting into either extreme end of the activity spectrum— either too little activity or too much. Neither is healthy for the patient with fatigue.

A second and perhaps even more important issue is how we reconcile ourselves to having less energy to do things in life. Many SSF members reported in the survey that they cut down on family or social activities (58 percent), limited physical activities (64 percent), and did less work around the house (64 percent). We live in a society where being productive is equated with success; it is very closely linked with our self-esteem. Unless we feel that we have something to contribute, we may begin to question our worth as human beings. We find ourselves being battered every day by our judgments about our productivity. Buying a birthday cake rather than making it at home can feel like a major transgression if we've been raised to believe that only homemade cakes are valued. Likewise, vacuuming every other week rather than weekly can prompt self-ridicule and accusations of being dirty, lazy, and inadequate. In the workplace, it can be just as bad. Reducing work hours or sales territory can create feelings of inadequacy and failure in an environment that is aggressively focused on bigger and more.

Dealing with this issue takes guts. It really means questioning our assumptions about what makes a person worthwhile and valuable. It involves scrutinizing our priorities and investing our limited energy in those activities that are most important to us. Yes, we could manage to bake and ice the birthday cake, but then we'd be too exhausted to enjoy the birthday party. Which is more important? Most of us would answer that it is spending enjoyable time with people we care about. So we'll need to do a lot of self-talk to assuage our guilt about the bakery cake in order to make the healthiest decision. When it comes to dealing with fatigue, all of the "shoulds" that we've acquired are the enemy. They are what drive us to try to do too much, because behind the "should" is the belief that if we don't, then either something awful will happen or (worse) we will be a worthless human being. These are incredibly powerful taskmasters. We need to muster the courage to question all of our "shoulds" and those that are imposed by our family, friends, and workplace. What we find when we do this is that many can be put aside or modified without dire consequences. Maintaining our self-esteem is the most important goal.

Pain

Many patients with Sjogren's experience chronic pain. Joint pain may be an effect of Sjogren's, or it may be due to the fact that many Sjogren's patients have an additional rheumatologic disorder such as rheumatoid arthritis, osteoarthritis, scleroderma, or fibromyalgia. Pain is one of the most distressing symptoms to experience. By definition it is very unpleasant and keeps intruding like a loud dog that won't stop barking. Patients with chronic pain describe how exhausting it can be to constantly struggle to cope with the pain. Dealing with pain for short bursts of time is difficult enough, but when it goes on for days, weeks, and longer, it can wear a person out. It is not surprising that patients with chronic pain consistently have higher rates of depression than patients with less or no pain. Earlier we noted that overall, 29 percent of SSF members reported depression as one of their most troubling symptoms. In fact, depression is significantly higher in SSF members with pain syndromes such as fibromyalgia (45 percent) and migraine headache (41 percent).

How we respond to pain can powerfully influence our total pain experience. Very early in our development, the occurrence of pain signals that some harm is being inflicted on our body and that we need to take immediate action to stop it. The young child who reaches out and touches something hot quickly withdraws her hand and learns that the pain signaled that her fingers were getting burned. When we burn our finger, scrape our knee falling off our bike, or stub our toe, each instance of pain is appropriately interpreted as harm coming to our body. Human beings have strong emotional reactions to pain and a strong instinct to avoid harm. The child who has fallen off her bike is crying as much from the surprise, fear, and embarrassment of the event as she is crying from the pain. To take the example a step farther, the more frightened and distressed she feels, the more pain she will feel.

The difficulty with chronic pain is that it doesn't always follow the simple rules learned as a child. Often chronic pain is not associated with an acute harm being directed toward the body that must be stopped immediately. For the vast majority of conditions associated with chronic pain, pulling away or stopping an activity will do little to stop the pain. Take fibromyalgia, for example, where it feels like awful things are happening in the muscles. The pain is not signaling harm to the muscles; rather, it appears that the pain is being generated by chemical imbalances in the nervous system. Dealing effectively with chronic pain starts with relearning the meaning of pain such that it no longer sets off the disaster alarm system in our mind. The sirens have to be turned off, the fear has to be quieted, and the catastrophizing has to be minimized. Instead of going with our first impulse—"Oh, no! This is terrible; I can't stand it. Please make it stop!"—we have to learn new ways of talking to ourselves. Recognizing the pain, registering disappointment, and then reassuring ourselves that we don't need to be alarmed set the stage for subsequent coping strategies that can considerably reduce the perception of pain and its impact on our life.

Managing Depression, Anger, Fatigue, and Pain

Approaches to Coping

Given the choice, no one would opt for coping with a chronic illness. Everyone would sign up for the cure. Modern medicine has dazzled us with cutting-edge breakthroughs in treating disease. Even something as deadly as AIDS has begun to submit to the clever strategies and healing tools of doctors. The National Institutes of Health spend billions of dollars every year researching cures for asthma, diabetes, heart disease, cancer, and many other diseases. The cure for Sjogren's syndrome, unfortunately, does not appear to be around the corner. Thus, when we are told that we need to learn to cope with an illness, it suggests that it's okay to settle for coping instead of pulling out all of the stops to eliminate the symptoms or the disease entirely. "Is my doctor really putting all of his energy into figuring out what is wrong with me and trying different things to help? Or once he realizes that it's a nonmalignant, chronic illness, does he lose interest and any motivation to keep exploring ways to help? Does anyone realize how incredibly hard it is to cope with all of these symptoms and the way it interferes with my life?"

In fact, we face all kinds of challenges throughout our lives that require us to cope with situations that we can't fix or "cure." Consider the challenge of financial problems, a stressful marriage, the death of a spouse or child, a gang-infested neighborhood, a difficult boss, ethnic or racial discrimination, or even difficult in-laws. Coping with situations that are far from optimal is an inescapable part of the human condition. Illness is just one of the greatest challenges for people who are otherwise blessed. However, there is no rule that says that an individual can't have many difficult challenges in life. It is not uncommon to see patients struggling with Sjogren's syndrome on top of a series of already very difficult life circumstances. For patients living in dangerous communities, or who have stressful, low-paying jobs, or whose family life is chaotic, there is a mountain of challenges to cope with. Life's unfairness comes in many shapes and sizes.

Researchers have been studying coping with daily hassles and large adversity for the last 30 years. Much has been learned during that time about what makes coping effective and what styles of coping are associated with poor outcome. There is also work that has been done that looks at patients' readiness to begin the process of coping. This research shows that patients are at different stages of readiness for coping. Some are well on their way, while others are still at the first stage where they only want to consider a cure and do not want to consider steps that they could take to manage their illness better. Where patients stand in terms of their readiness for adaptive coping is in part tied to their state of mind: how much of their energy is still going into anger and how depressed they are. Both anger and depression are states of mind that interfere with the view that we can be calm, accepting, and empowered to achieve a good quality of life in spite of life's challenges. When we feel like a wronged party, a victim, we seek to blame and to demand justice and restitution. When we are depressed, our sadness, pessimism, lack of energy, and helplessness undercut our ability to think positively and creatively about ways to adapt. Effective coping with Sjogren's requires first a self-assessment of the state of our anger and mood. Both need to be brought within healthy limits, or the impact of our illness on our well-being is going to continue to be negative.

In the section on depression, we noted that many Sjogren's patients are depressed and that the side effects of antidepressant medications may be intolerable because they increase dryness. Fortunately, medication is not the only way to successfully treat depression. One option that we mentioned is psychological therapy. Indeed, research has shown that some types of psychological therapy can be just as effective as medication for treating depression: cognitive-behavioral therapy and interpersonal therapy. Each of these treatments helps the patient to break the negative spiral of social withdrawal and losing interest in pleasurable activities. Cognitive-behavioral therapy helps patients to think about themselves and their situations in ways that are more positive. A shift to thinking about the cup as half full rather than half empty is a simple example of this. Reducing the maladaptive coping pattern called "catastrophizing" is an especially important cognitive change for Sjogren's patients and those with other chronic diseases. Research clearly shows that patients who come to dire conclusions about their situation have a much poorer outcome than those who do less catastrophizing. Interpersonal therapy addresses the functioning of our interpersonal relationships, which are so important to our feeling positively about ourselves and our lives. Therapy that focuses on improving and enriching our interpersonal experiences can have a dramatic effect on depression.

Physical exercise has also been shown to have positive effects on mood and well-being. Although it is not recommended as a primary treatment for clinical depression, it can be a very important component of an overall approach to reducing depression. Moreover, physical exercise has so many other positive benefits. There is another negative spiral very common in medical patients, called deconditioning. Pain, stiffness, and fatigue are all compelling reasons that cause patients to shy away from physical activity. However, as patients do less activity, stiffness, pain, fatigue, and sleep problems actually increase. The body becomes deconditioned—that is, weak and out of shape. The more deconditioning sets in, the worse patients feel and the less likely they are to be active. It is not uncommon for patients to explain that they know they should be more active, but every time they are, they feel that they pay a heavy price for the next few days with aches and exhaustion. For them, exercise seems to only make things worse. Patients who report this are not lazy or whiners; rather, they are describing a common problem that requires some expert guidance to solve. Unless patients know what types of activity or exercise are appropriate for their particular condition and how much to do, many will fail. Patients with joint disease, such as rheumatoid arthritis, osteoarthritis, or fibromyalgia, can aggravate their illness with the wrong forms of exercise. Many patients have to start out very slowly and very gradually build up their stamina and endurance.

Likewise, knowing which exercises are best and which to avoid makes all the difference in starting and maintaining a successful reconditioning program. Physical therapists are trained to design individualized programs for patients, to continuously reassess progress, and to work out difficulties that emerge along the way. This type of professional guidance can be the difference between demoralizing failure and success for many patients.

A less individualized approach, but much better than trying to figure it out on your own, is the Arthritis Foundation's People with Arthritis Can Exercise (PACE) classes. PACE is a group exercise program led by trained instructors that uses gentle activities to help increase joint flexibility and range of motion and to help maintain muscle strength and increase overall stamina. A second program available through the local chapters is the Arthritis Foundation's Aquatic Program. Since water provides buoyancy and protects the joints from impact, it is especially comfortable for patients with arthritis pain and stiffness. Like the PACE program, it takes patients through a series of gentle exercises to increase flexibility, strength, and stamina. Reversing the deconditioning spiral can be one of the most important steps a patient can take to improve the quality of their life. More information about these programs is available at www.arthritis.org.

Communicating Needs

Human beings have a deep need to share their experiences and to feel understood. Communication weaves our life journey with those around us. It is a fundamental way of helping us to make sense of our experiences and to have others recognize and validate those experiences. When we listen to ourselves speak out loud, we sometimes gain a different perspective about events compared with listening to the private, internal dialogue in our head. Plus, the reactions and comments of those we are speaking to provide further input into our evolving view of the experience and its meaning for us.

Communication is fundamental to the day-to-day human experience. But not all communication is effective or successful. It can break down at lots of points along the way. It can start with ineffective delivery of the information, and it can continue with woefully inept listening. In all cases, ineffective communication is a source of distress and a frequent precipitant of disappointment and interpersonal conflict. How is it that such a vital aspect of successful living is often done so poorly? Probably because we've never been explicitly taught good communication and listening skills. It is not an accident that many corporations spend thousands of dollars sending their executives and managers to communication training programs. They can have a great product or service, but if they don't know how to convey that to their potential customers in a convincing way, they won't get sales. Furthermore, if they don't know how to listen to what their customers are describing about their particular needs, they can't address these issues and sell more product.

Good communication is no less important for Sjogren's patients. We need to be able to tell people what is happening to us, how we are feeling, and what we need. The more important an experience is to us, the greater our need to share it. Like other patients with a chronic illness, Sjogren's can become a central focus of our lives. We are trying to understand it and to master it. When we talk about it with others, we are no longer alone with it. Our emotions such as pain, fear, and anger are recognized, and our struggle is validated. Joining the Sjogren's Syndrome Foundation and participating in the activities of local chapters and support groups can help. It opens up opportunities to hear that others will help us or at least that they sympathize with us. When we communicate effectively, we inform others of what we are or are not able to do and why. And not least of all, good communication equips us with the ability to specifically ask for what we need. We need to be direct—it's a mistake to assume that other people can read our mind.

Sjogren's syndrome presents special issues for communication. Sometimes we sense that our comments and complaints are becoming old and tiresome for our friends and family. Basically, we worry that they don't want to hear about it anymore. There is nothing new to be said and nothing new to be done. But if we struggle along quietly in order not to create discomfort in the people around us, we may create a sense of isolation for ourselves. However, recognizing that our illness creates distress in those who care about us can help us to solve this communication dilemma.

Most of us tend to respond to difficulties by problem solving; this is particularly true for men. But none of us likes to feel helpless and inept at solving the problem. At this point in time, Sjogren's syndrome is a chronic problem that can't be totally solved. It is going to persist and perhaps even worsen over time. Not a happy affair for the problem solver! What we need to realize and then communicate is that often we are not expecting anyone to solve the problem. We may be feeling particularly bad today and just want to whine and complain a little, so that we are not alone with the experience. Sometimes we are just looking for some sympathy—a little extra love and concern as a salve for the hurt. All of this serves to keep us from feeling alone and to be reassured that we are important and loved by others and that they will continue to stick by us. So if these are the things that we are really looking for when we talk about our illness, we need to let people off the hook of trying to make it better for us; instead, we should let them just listen and give us support. Many of the people in our life will be willing to do this.

Communication with our health care professionals is a special case. We have a limited amount of time with them, we have several of them (rheumatologist, dentist, ophthalmologist, etc.), we may feel intimidated, and often we have hefty expectations about their ability to solve our problems. It is no wonder that Sjogren's patients often leave their doctor's office upset by what did not happen.

The intersection between patient and doctor that is problematic is when the patient has expectations for the doctor that are not reasonable. Doctors are limited by the boundaries of current medical science, and medical science has limitless frontiers of yet undiscovered knowledge. What this means for Sjogren's patients is that our doctors are not going to know precisely what is causing our dryness and other associated symptoms. Although it is frustrating to us, they may have to watch a symptom over weeks, months, or years to generate confidence in their interpretation of its meaning for our health. And they may never figure out what to do about it. Patients' responses to many treatments still resemble a game of chance: some patients will improve, others will show no response, while others will suffer serious side effects. If we want a healthy, productive relationship with our doctor, we need to have reasonable expectations. We have to be willing to accept that our doctor may not know and may have little or nothing in his tool kit to help. At the same time, we need to be educated and informed consumers and be on top of possible new treatments.

The next time you have an appointment with your doctor, try the following. Before you go, imagine leaving the doctor's office having had a very successful visit. What about the visit was pleasing? Did he or she spend some extra time with you so you could get through many of your questions? Did he express empathy for the rough time you've been having? Did he give you some suggestions about ways of managing your symptoms so you can get more done and feel more comfortable? Did he reassure you? Was he willing to talk with you without getting irritated about the magnet therapy you were thinking of trying or a new herb that you heard about? Did he agree to talk with your other doctors to keep your medical care better coordinated? Remember that your agenda and that of your doctor are not necessarily in sync when you enter the exam room, and doctors are no better at mind reading than anyone else. Once you've identified what made the imagined visit a success for you, then consider what steps you can take to make it happen. Clear, direct communication with your doctor about what you need from the visit will increase the likelihood of success. If you don't ask, it's going to be hard to get what you want. On the other hand, if after a few visits with your doctor, you are still leaving the office dissatisfied, then you have to do some soul-searching about your style and expectations or you need to consider whether another doctor would form a more satisfying partnership with you.

Take Control

In 1977, Dr. Albert Bandura, a psychologist at Stanford University, introduced what has become a very important concept in the management of chronic illness. The concept, self-efficacy, refers to a person's belief in his or her ability to exert control over important aspects of life, as opposed to having to passively accept things as they are. Like most personal characteristics, individuals vary in how much of the characteristic they have. Over the past 25 years, research has focused on the impact of self-efficacy in patients with chronic illness, especially rheumatologic diseases. The studies have repeatedly come up with the same result: the greater the sense of self-efficacy, that is, the ability to reduce symptoms and disability, the lower the ratings of pain, fatigue, depression, disability, and so on. What is fascinating is that the research suggests that patients higher on self-efficacy are not necessarily doing anything different, such as exercising or pacing, compared with patients with lower self-efficacy. Rather, it appears that having a mind-set of empowerment over adversity rather than a mind-set of victimization can contribute to greater well-being in these patients.

Let's take a very salient example. Dryness is a noxious experience, one that readily creates feelings of being trapped and victimized by those suffering with it morning, noon, and night. For the patient with little self-efficacy, the belief is that only medication or a cure can lessen the extreme discomfort, and they have little choice but to endure it. Such patients believe that nothing they do will make any difference. Compare this with the Sjogren's patient who has a take-charge attitude, who keeps trying different strategies to see what helps, and who knows that once the doctors or nurses have done their job, then the patient's job of effectively managing their illness is just beginning. In the field of pain, research has discovered that many factors come into play to determine how much pain a patient experiences. The mind-body connection is really at work with pain as well as many other symptoms. How we talk to ourselves about our pain, how we emotionally react to our pain, and how we alter our behavior in response to pain ultimately play a large part in how much pain we experience. Similarly, how we react to dryness plays a large part in how much it interferes with our functioning. The key issue is the extent to which we feel that we can have some control over our symptoms and disability. The more we accept responsibility, then the less passive and victimized we will be, and the more likely we are to make important and effective contributions to our health and well-being.

Summing Up

The mind-body relationship is extremely important in patients with Sjogren's syndrome and can affect patient perception of fatigue, pain, and other symptoms. Development of more effective psychosocial coping strategies can greatly alleviate symptoms and improves patient quality of life.

Swamy Venuturupalli, MD

19 Complementary and Alternative Therapies for Sjogren's Syndrome

SJOGREN'S SYNDROME is a chronic autoimmune condition characterized by the sicca syndrome complex. Oftentimes Sjogren's is associated with other autoimmune disorders such as rheumatoid arthritis (RA) and systemic lupus erythematosus (SLE). An estimated 35–50 percent of patients with Sjogren's have an inflammatory arthritis similar to rheumatoid arthritis, and approximately 50 percent of patients have symptoms suggestive of fibromyalgia (a chronic pain syndrome with significant muscle soreness).

In this chapter, a review of the available evidence to support the use of complementary and alternative medicine (CAM) for Sjogren's syndrome is presented. An extensive search of the scientific literature yielded very few clinical studies dealing with Sjogren's syndrome specifically. Hence, a significant part of this chapter will focus on the use of CAM for arthritis and fibromyalgia, both very common associations in Sjogren's syndrome.

Complementary and alternative medicine refers to a wide array of therapies that are not generally learned in conventional medical training or used in conventional medical practice. In the last decade these therapies have become extremely popular, with about 40 percent of Americans using CAM for chronic conditions, at an estimated annual expenditure of $27 billion per year. Patients with rheumatic diseases perhaps use CAM at a rate greater than for all other diseases.

Several important issues and concerns arise with the use of CAM by patients:

1 A lot of these therapies, even though considered natural, are not free of side effects and toxicity.

2 Since a lot of these medications are manufactured without proper regulation, there may be undeclared additions and adulterations to the medicines.

3 The authenticity of the claimed ingredients is a huge question mark.

4 There is a possibility of severe interactions between prescribed medicine and CAM.

5 There are several behavioral patterns associated with CAM, such as medication discontinuation, use of CAM with no professional supervision, and a low willingness to report CAM side effects on the part of patients and practitioners that may adversely affect patient health.

With this background, the following therapies will be discussed for their relevance to rheumatic diseases:

Dietary therapies

Herbal therapies and nutriceuticals

Manual and manipulative therapies

Acupuncture

Ayurveda and yoga

CAM therapies specific for Sjogren's syndrome

Diet and Dietary Therapies

Panush and colleagues reviewed the scientific literature on diet and dietary therapies for rheumatic conditions in an issue of *Rheumatic Disease Clinics of North America*. The following is a summary of the major studies reviewed and presented in that publication.

Fasting

Fasting has been proposed as a therapy for rheumatic conditions. Several clinical trials have shown that fasting improved symptoms of rheumatic disease in some patients. For example, 5 of 15 patients with rheumatoid arthritis who fasted for 7 to 10 days showed improvement, compared with only 1 of 10 controls in one study. Another prospective study investigated the effects of complete fasting on patients with RA. Forty-three patients underwent a fast, consisting only of water, that lasted seven days. Both objective and subjective symptoms showed significant improvement. Thus, fasting may improve rheumatic conditions. This improvement might be a result of weight loss and malnutrition, which can suppress immunity. Fasting in a Sjogren's patient, however, can exacerbate dryness due to dehydration.

Elimination or Exclusion Diets

Exclusion or elimination diets are used to detect foods that are suspected of causing food allergies and thus triggering attacks of illness. Suspected foods are avoided for a specified period of time to clear the system and are then reintroduced in a carefully controlled sequence. Symptoms that reappear are thought to be a reaction to particular foods. These foods are then eliminated from the diet for a considerable time.

Several studies have been conducted to determine whether sensitivity to certain foods can exacerbate RA symptoms. For example, Darlington and colleagues reported that some patients with rheumatoid arthritis benefited from the elimination of certain foods, including corn, wheat, pork, bacon, orange juice, milk, oats, rye, eggs, beef, coffee, malt, cheese, grapefruit, tomato, butter, sugar, and soy, in descending order of frequency. These patients experienced symptomatic deterioration with the reintroduction of these foods. None of these studies has been rigorously controlled, and therefore none can be interpreted as being definitive.

More recent studies by Panush and colleagues gave patients blinded food challenges of food in capsule form. Only 3 of 16 patients convincingly demonstrated an increase in subjective and objective rheumatologic symptoms when they were challenged in this blinded manner with foods that they claimed to be allergic to.

Based on a review of all the available evidence, it appears that only a small number of rheumatoid arthritis patients clearly demonstrate food-related allergies. These patients will benefit from the elimination of these foods from their diet.

Elemental or Hypoallergenic Diets

Elemental diets contain no complex protein or peptides, but do contain free amino acids, which are components of the proteins and the peptides. In some experiences in the published literature, elemental diets appear to be beneficial. For example, in the study by Panush and colleagues in which patients were challenged with allergens in a double-blind fashion, most patients showed improvement on an elemental diet, suggesting that there may be a role for this diet in treating rheumatic conditions.

Dietary Supplements

Ginger has been used for many years in Ayurveda (the traditional Indian medical system) and other healing traditions. In an open trial of 28 patients, ginger was shown to be effective in reducing inflammatory symptoms.

Bromelain is an enzyme derived from the pineapple plant. There is no clinical evidence to support the use of bromelain for rheumatic conditions.

Collagen type II was studied in a multicenter, double-blind, placebo-controlled trial. There was no efficacy associated with the use of collagen type II for rheumatoid arthritis patients in this trial.

Shark cartilage has been suggested as a treatment for osteoarthritis, rheumatoid arthritis, and lupus, but there are no adequate clinical trials to substantiate the use of shark cartilage.

The higher susceptibility of women to autoimmune conditions has suggested a role for sex steroids in these diseases. Low serum levels of *dehydroepiandrosterone (DHEA)* have been measured in postmenopausal women with RA, men with RA, and patients with SLE. DHEA has been preliminarily studied in RA and Sjogren's, but did not show any efficacy. Research is currently being conducted on the use of DHEA in SLE, and these studies show a lot of promise in controlling the symptoms of SLE. DHEA is not without side effects, which include prostate enlargement in men and masculinization or liver damage in women, increased risk for heart disease, insulin resistance, and uterine and other hormone influenced cancers. Hence, if DHEA is being used for rheumatic diseases, it needs to be done in proper dosing under the guidance of a physician.

Vitamin and Nutritional Therapies

Antioxidants such as vitamin A, C, and E have been studied for their role in preventing oxidative tissue damage and in preventing rheumatic diseases. Low levels of beta-carotene (the precursor to vitamin A) were found in the blood of rheumatoid arthritis patients compared with controls. However, no study of the administration of vitamin A to RA patients has been done. Vitamin A deficiency can cause dry eye but is seldom detected among people with Sjogren's.

In randomized control trials, vitamin E was found to be as effective as diclofenac, which is a nonsteroidal anti-inflammatory drug, and more effective than placebo in reducing symptoms of rheumatoid arthritis.

Ascorbic acid or vitamin C has been found at low levels in the blood of RA patients, but there is no convincing clinical data for its use in rheumatoid arthritis, or other rheumatic disorders.

Dietary Fatty Acids

Omega-3 and omega-6 fatty acids have been found to have several anti-inflammatory properties. Eicosapentaenoic acid is an omega-3 fatty acid found in cold-water fish. Gamma-linolenic acid is an omega-3 fatty acid found in large quantities in plant seed oils such as flaxseed oil, borage seed oil, and evening primrose oil.

The clinical usefulness of fish oils and plant-derived fatty acids has been studied in multiple clinical trials. A review of all these clinical trials suggest that fish oil is superior to placebo for improving joint tenderness and morning stiffness in rheumatoid arthritis patients. Flaxseed oil showed initial benefit in RA patients, but after three months of follow-up, no beneficial improvements were demonstrated.

Polyunsaturated fatty acids have not been consistently beneficial in the treatment of SLE. Fish oil has been shown to be useful in patients with Raynaud's phenomenon and in some patients of rheumatoid arthritis.

Thus, fish oil and plant seed oils may have modest benefits at best in rheumatic conditions. Fish oil supplements, unlike whole fish, typically do not contain any mercury, and can be taken in anti-inflammatory dosages without problems.

Herbal Anti-inflammatory Medications

Herbal medications are exceedingly popular for a variety of conditions. Between 1990 and 1997 use of herbal medicines increased by 400 percent in the United States. A large proportion of these are used for rheumatologic conditions. While a lot of patients believe that herbal medicines are safer than pharmaceuticals, this is not always the case.

The use of herbal therapies may give rise to significant side effects and interactions with prescribed medications. Moreover, since the manufacture of herbal supplements is not well regulated, the potency of herbs may vary from batch to batch, and this could give rise to many additional problems. Having said this, it appears that the incidence of adverse effects from herbal therapies is fairly low.

Most of the herbs used as anti-inflammatories seem to affect the cyclooxygenase and lipooxygenase pathways, which are pathways that cause inflammation in the body. These are the same pathways that are targeted by nonsteroidal anti-inflammatory drugs such as aspirin, ibuprofen, celecoxib, and so on. Other pathways that reduce inflammatory mediators have also been shown to be affected favorably. Herbal medications may have weaker inhibition of inflammatory pathways compared with synthetic drugs. Thus, herbal anti-inflammatory medications, while not as potent as synthetic drugs, may have fewer adverse effects than pharmaceuticals. In acute and severe pain, herbs are probably less helpful than pharmaceuticals, but may have a role to play in milder and more chronic pain.

Recently, a systematic review of the scientific literature described 19 randomized controlled trials. Encouraging data was found for evening primrose oil, borage seed oil, devil's claw, Phytodolor (a commercially available mixture of herbs), and willow bark extract.

Evening Primrose Oil

Evening primrose oil contains GLA (gamma-linoleic acid) and eicosapentaenoic acid, which are anti-inflammatory fatty acids. In a well-conducted clinical trial evening primrose oil was found to be superior to placebo for osteoarthritis. Side effects reported were nausea and rash. Patients who are on antipsychotic medications should avoid this because of increased risk of seizures. The recommended dose is 500–1,500 mg of GLA.

Borage Seed Oil

Borage seed oil contains GLA. Two randomized, placebo-controlled trials showed significant improvement in arthritis with its use. Negligible side effects were reported in the trials. A dose of 1–2 grams has a potentially toxic amount of pyrazolidine alkaloids, and patients on antiepileptic drugs should avoid it because of increased seizure risk.

Devil's Claw

This is a very popular herb used for inflammatory conditions. The active principle is harpagoside. Two randomized, controlled trials showed positive results in acute low back pain patients. Two other randomized, controlled trials showed positive results in osteoarthritis patients. The recommended dose is up to 9 grams per day for three to four months. Significant gastrointestinal toxicity may occur, and it is contraindicated in patients with ulcer disease. Also, it is contraindicated in patients who are on the anticoagulant warfarin, because devil's claw increases in the level of warfarin in the blood.

Phytodolor

Phytodolor is a commercially available product from Germany. A dose of 100 ml contains the following herbs: *Populus tremula* 60 ml, *Fraxmus excelsior* 20 ml, and *Solidago vergaurea* 20 ml. There are four randomized controlled trials on rheumatic pain of all sorts, with a total of 225 patients. All four studies showed a significant decrease in pain compared with placebo. The therapeutic dosage is 30–40 drops three times a day. No significant adverse reactions have been reported.

Willow Bark Extract

The active ingredient in willow bark is salicin (an aspirin-like compound). Two randomized, controlled trials showed benefit in osteoarthritis patients compared with placebo. However, there are many possible side effects, including exacerbation of asthma, allergic rhinitis, contact dermatitis, salicylate toxicity, and liver and kidney damage. This drug also interacts with many other medications; for example, it increases levels of phenytoin (an anti-epileptic) and warfarin (a blood thinner).

Acupuncture

Acupuncture is a component of traditional Chinese health care and can be traced back 2,000 years. The general theory of acupuncture is based on the premise that there are patterns of energy that flow through the body that are essential for health. Acupuncture is believed to correct imbalances of energy or *qi* as it flows through 12 primary meridians (channels) and 8 extraordinary meridians. Practitioners may use heat, pressure, friction, suction, electric stimulation, and lasers in addition to the traditional needles that are placed on specific points in the affected meridians.

Acupuncture has been studied in clinical trials for the treatment of osteoarthritis (degenerative arthritis), rheumatoid arthritis, fibromyalgia, and back pain. One of the significant problems in studying acupuncture in randomized clinical trials is the designing of a placebo arm, where controlled acupuncture needs to be given to patients without them knowing that they are in a placebo group. This significant design issue makes the study of acupuncture very difficult, and hence very few good clinical trials have been conducted. Having said that, there appears to be fairly good evidence that acupuncture is better for back pain than sham or placebo acupuncture. There is only one good trial that has studied acupuncture for fibromyalgia in a scientifically sound way, and this trial shows that acupuncture may help. There is only one good randomized trial using acupuncture for rheumatoid arthritis, and again, this shows that acupuncture may be helpful. For the pain of osteoarthritis of the knee, there is strong evidence that acupuncture is better than sham acupuncture.

There is no clear-cut evidence that the use of acupuncture improves a patient's ability to function (as opposed to improving the symptom of pain). Thus acupuncture may be used as an adjunct when dealing with pain from any of the above conditions.

Ayurvedic Medicine

The term *Ayurveda* is a Sanskrit word that translates as "knowledge of life or longevity" and refers to the ancient Indian system of medicine. This is a comprehensive system that incorporates its own theory of illness, pathogenesis of different conditions, and a therapeutic pharmaco-poeia that includes several hundred herbs and thousands of combinations of these herbs. Therapeutics in Ayurveda are multifaceted and include diet, yoga and other exercise therapies, mental relaxation techniques, and herbal therapies along with purification therapies.

Ayurveda is still practiced in India and is now becoming increasingly popular in the West. Ayurvedic theory of disease is based on the *tridosha* theory, which holds that the body contains three humors or *doshas* called *vata, pitta,* and *kapha. Vata* is involved with psychomotor activities, *pitta* with metabolism, and *kapha* with structural integrity of the body. Each person is believed to have a unique combination of *vata, pitta,* and *kapha* in the body at the time of birth. This combination changes as the person progresses through life. When there is an abnormal accumulation or deficiency of one or more doshas in one's body, disease is thought to result. Ayurvedic therapies are usually aimed at restoring the balance of these three *doshas* to the original unique combination of each person.

Numerous herbs have been described in Ayurvedic literature to possess antirheumatic activity. Unfortunately, clinical trials of these are far and few between. In one randomized clinical trial, Kulkarni and colleagues studied a combination of four Ayurvedic herbs in osteoarthritis patients. These included *Withania somnifera, Boswellia serrata, Curcuma longa,* and zinc ash. The patients on the Ayurvedic herbal combination did significantly better than the placebo group. In another trial, Chopra and colleagues studied two Ayurvedic formulas, RA-1 and RA-11, in rheumatoid arthritis patients. Again, these herbs resulted in significant improvement in symptoms compared with placebo.

Ayurvedic medicine holds a lot of promise for treating a number of conditions. Intriguingly, Ayurvedic medicine strongly believes in a connection between the gut and rheumatic conditions, something that has been validated more recently by Western science in conditions such as ankylosing spondylitis and other disorders. A lot of the herbs that are thought to be active against arthritis have not been validated in randomized clinical trials. This is clearly something that needs to be done. Moreover, Ayurvedic herbs suffer from the same problem as other herbal medications, namely, lack of standardization and lack of quality regulation. The use, development, and scientific validation of Ayurvedic herbs is certainly a very important potential source of future treatments for rheumatic conditions.

Yoga

Yoga is a complete system of spiritual and physical pursuit that aims to unite the body with the mind. This system developed many thousands of years ago in India and is still practiced today. The popular form of yoga in the West is hatha yoga, which emphasizes certain postures. Hatha yoga, "the yoga of activity," addresses the body and mind and requires discipline and effort. In addition to the postures, yoga includes an entire philosophy of life. Thus, yoga is meant to be practiced in the larger context of a spiritual discipline. Large numbers of Americans are practicing yoga for its proposed health benefits.

As a therapy, yoga is a system designed to refine human physiology. Postures or *asanas,* if done properly, are believed to affect every gland and organ in the body. Postures have to be adjusted to position various organs, joints, and bones properly so that the desired physiologic changes may occur. Distribution of the body weight has to be even on the joints and muscles so that there is no injury. Therapeutic yoga is a performance of postures for treating medical disorders.

A review of the evidence that is published about yoga shows a few positive clinical trials. References to clinical trials in asthma, hypertension, pain management, diabetes, and mood have been found. However, the quality of most of these studies is not very good.

In the rheumatic diseases, two small, controlled, but non-double-blind studies performed by Garfinkel and colleagues show promise for the use of yoga in osteoarthritis of the fingers and carpal tunnel syndrome.

There are certain risks to yoga treatment, which may include flaring of rheumatic conditions if proper precautions are not taken. For example, for persons with arthritis, a posture should be developed slowly, with as little strain on the inflamed joints and muscles as possible. Choosing an appropriate yoga instructor is certainly a challenge, and this itself limits its use as a therapeutic modality for arthritis.

Alternative Therapies Specifically for Sjogren's Syndrome

A search of the scientific literature on CAM therapies for Sjogren's syndrome resulted in only five published articles. In a study by Johansson and colleagues, mouth rinses with the linseed extract salinum were studied in a controlled, double-blind manner. The use of salinum with or without chlorhexidine (an antimicrobial substance) was shown to reduce oral bacterial counts, oral dryness, and symptoms of speaking problems and oral burning. Thus the salinum may be useful in reducing oral symptoms in patients with Sjogren's syndrome.

In another study, Longo Vital, an herb-based tablet enriched with vitamins, was studied in patients with Sjogren's syndrome and compared with placebo. The authors showed that Longo Vital may have a modest effect on clinical and immunoinflammatory markers in Sjogren's syndrome.

Lastly, List and colleagues studied acupuncture in treating patients with primary Sjogren's syndrome. The authors were not able to show any statistically significant differences between the acupuncture group and the control group in unstimulated salivary secretion and most subjective variables. Based on this study, acupuncture cannot be recommended to patients for symptoms of oral or eye dryness.

Summing Up

In this broad overview of common CAM therapies for Sjogren's syndrome I have not reviewed several common therapies, such as manual and manipulative therapies, since they are mainly useful for symptomatic relief from pain syndromes and may have limited relevance to Sjogren's syndrome patients. Traditional Chinese medicine and other traditional healing systems have not been dealt with in significant detail; this would be beyond the scope of this chapter. Cited and additional references are available by contacting swamy_ucla@yahoo.com.

Based on a review of CAM for Sjogren's and related disorders, it is clear that CAM may play a positive role in managing Sjogren's symptoms, arthritis, and fibromyalgia. Finding a qualified CAM professional is not always easy, and neither is finding high-quality CAM products. Most patients find it hard to communicate about CAM with their health care professionals, but they must attempt to do so, because the potential for adverse interactions between conventional medicines and CAM is a risk that should be minimized.

20 How Are Drugs Tested for Sjogren's?

RELATIVELY FEW DRUGS HAVE been thoroughly tested for the treatment of Sjogren's syndrome. Current treatment for Sjogren's is aimed at the symptoms, inflammation and complications of the disease. While a number of preparations are available for treating the complications of Sjogren's, such as those for yeast infections, which can exacerbate problems with mouth or vaginal dryness, and compounds for treatment of dry itchy skin, these medications and products were not expressively tested and approved for Sjogren's. Thus far, the only drugs approved for Sjogren's are for the dry mouth and dry eye symptoms of the disease. These drugs mark a major step forward in treating Sjogren's patients. However, few drugs to treat Sjogren's systemically have been tested, and no definitive evidence is available at this time showing that drugs that target the immune system are beneficial in Sjogren's.

Why Have So Few Drugs Been Tested for the Treatment of Sjogren's?

Aspects of the disease have hampered drug development. First, the lack of unanimity on diagnostic criteria for Sjogren's discouraged investigators in academia and the pharmaceutical industry from testing new treatments for the disease. However, published criteria for classifying cases as Sjogren's are very similar and vary mainly in their stringency. Closer agreement has emerged in recent years on diagnostic criteria and has resulted in the publication of revised classification criteria by the American-European Consensus Group. In addition, the disease has been perceived as being mild and not life-threatening. Thus, there has been a reluctance to use, test, or develop more powerful drugs in individuals with Sjogren's, because of concerns that the hazards of treatment would outweigh the potential benefits. Also, the best measures to assess the response of the disease to treatment have not been well characterized yet.

Over the past few years, meetings have been held to develop consensus on the optimal outcome measures for Sjogren's. This has resulted in a candidate set of outcome measures and a framework for their validation. Typically, clinical trials of Sjogren's have used measures that included symptoms of dryness and fatigue, objective measures of dry eye, such as the Schirmer test, van Bijsterveld score (a test for ocular dryness using a dye), or tear breakup time; objective measures of oral dryness such as stimulated or unstimulated salivary flow rates; and blood tests such as the erythrocyte sedimentation rate (ESR or sed rate) and the level of immunoglobulin G. In addition, the Short Form 36 (SF-36), a 36-item questionnaire that measures health-related quality of life, has been considered. Considerable work lies ahead in the validation of outcome measures in Sjogren's.

What Does Participation in a Clinical Trial Entail?

In part, what participation involves is related to the nature of the drug, biologic, or device that is being tested. It is also related to the phase of testing, which will be discussed below. A trial will usually involve a screening process that may begin with a telephone conversation. A screening visit is usually scheduled to determine whether or not a potential participant meets the criteria for inclusion in the study. For example, the investigators who designed the trial may require that a patient with Sjogren's also has a positive test for anti-Ro/SSA, even though a negative test does not preclude a diagnosis of Sjogren's. Also, it is important to be sure that a subject does not have any of the exclusion criteria, such as pregnancy. Usually the screening visit will involve completing questionnaires, a physical examination, blood tests, and sometimes X-rays or other radiological tests. In some cases, biopsies may be required. Before entering into a clinical trial, it is key to understand what the study is about, what treatment subjects will actually receive, and a clear and realistic assessment of the risks involved in the study. These issues should be presented in a clear manner in the informed-consent document that all prospective subjects are asked to read and sign if they agree to participate in the study.

How Are the Interests of Human Subjects Participating in Clinical Trials Protected?

Clinical research protocols must be reviewed by institutional review boards (IRBs) to determine the level of risk of the investigation or clinical trial, and to ensure that the participants have been adequately informed of the likely and possible risks of the study through informed-consent documents. IRBs ensure that the investigators comply with the regulations regarding clinical research. Typically, after the initial review, the study must undergo continuing review at intervals (at least annually) determined by the IRBs. An IRB is generally composed of individuals with experience in the disease under investigation, such as physicians, dentists, and psychologists. In addition, a biostatistician may be helpful in assessing that the information obtained from the study will be useful and will justify the participation of human subjects. However, there are often scientific review committees in research organizations to ensure that the design of the clinical trial is sound. In addition, one or more lay persons serve on the IRB to advocate for participants. They provide very useful input on the questions that participants might have and in ensuring that the informed-consent document will be well understood by the target population for the trial.

What Is the General Process for the Development and Testing of New Drugs?

The development of new treatments for various diseases is extremely complex and usually involves an understanding of the mechanisms of the disease. Basic science laboratory and animal studies often test hypotheses about the mechanisms of diseases. Then particular molecules may be targeted to block a deleterious process or augment a favorable process. The dominant paradigm is that of bringing a new treatment from the basic science laboratory bench to patients ("bench to bedside"). However, it is clear that the reverse also occurs, in that problems confronting clinicians may lead to basic science investigations of the mechanisms. Also, drugs that are approved for the treatment of one disease may serendipitously be found to be useful in an unrelated disease. This may prompt the formal investigation of the treatment in clinical trials.

New drugs may be developed from preclinical laboratory investigations and animal studies. Existing drugs may already have been developed, tested, and approved for the treatment of other diseases before being considered for Sjogren's. In some cases special large-scale industrial robotic systems are used to synthesize thousands of new compounds. Compounds may also be extracted from plants, fungi, bacteria, or other sources. In some settings a very large number of compounds may be screened by placing them into contact with cell line suspensions to develop a profile of their biological effects, which would suggest potential applications for the drugs.

Once these drugs have been identified, a much slower process is undertaken. Usually, the Food and Drug Administration (FDA) is consulted very early in the drug development process, since the FDA may require preclinical studies that have not been considered by the drug developers. Preclinical studies in animals allow for the determination of the drug's safety and biological mechanisms of action. Dosing studies can be performed in animals to determine the likely dose for humans. Prior to any clinical studies in humans, the FDA is consulted again before researchers file an investigational new drug application. The purpose of this meeting with the FDA is to resolve any preclinical issues and to ensure that the details of the drug development process for subsequent phases of drug development will be acceptable to the agency. After this, the drug development process will follow several phases. The general process is specified in the Code of Federal Regulations. By and large, drug development within industry tends to be on a "go/no-go" basis. At each step, safety, feasibility, and cost have to be considered, and many drugs do not progress beyond the early investigations. When failed drugs are included, the cost of bringing a single new drug to market may be in the hundreds of millions of dollars.

In the early stages, feasibility assessments take into account the prevalence of the disease (the number of existing cases in the population) and its incidence (the number of new cases per population per unit of time, e.g., cases per 100,000 population per year), since rare diseases may not allow a pharmaceutical company sufficient return to cover the costs of development. In addition, careful attention is given to the design of the human clinical trials to ensure that valid answers to important questions, appropriate to each phase of development, are obtained. A protocol is written outlining the background data motivating testing of the drug, the study design, the rationale for the number of subjects to be enrolled in the study, what measures will be used to determine the success or failure of the treatment, how potential adverse events will be monitored, how the data will be managed and analyzed, what will be done during subjects' visits, a copy of the informed consent document, and other considerations pertinent to the trial. This protocol undergoes scientific, IRB, and other reviews. For each phase of development, protocols must be written, and various reviews are required. The developmental phases are outlined below.

Phase I: Dose and Safety Testing

Phase I testing usually involves 20 to 100 subjects. An idea of the safety and appropriate dosing levels has already been obtained in animals. Here subjects are treated with low doses that are increased carefully. If adverse events are observed at a particular dose, higher doses are usually not tried. Studies of how the drug is absorbed, metabolized, and cleared in humans give a more comprehensive picture of the drug. Although animal studies may have suggested the drug may be useful in treating particular disease processes, no attempt is made in Phase I studies to determine whether the treatment works.

Phase II: Further Assessment of Safety in a Larger Number of Patients and Evidence of Efficacy

Phase II studies usually involve 100 to 300 subjects. *Efficacy* refers to whether a drug is able to successfully treat a condition and is usually determined under controlled conditions. It should be distinguished from *effectiveness*, which is evaluated among patients in the real world and is usually determined after a drug is already on the market. Phase II investigations allow drugs that have emerged from Phase I studies with an acceptable safety profile to be further tested for safety. The data from the Phase II study are used to calculate the number of patients required to establish safety and efficacy in the pivotal Phase III study.

Phase III: Proof of Efficacy and Further Safety Testing

Phase III usually involves 300 to 1,000 subjects. During this phase determination of efficacy is of major importance. Many disorders are not sufficiently common to allow a Phase III study to be performed at one center. Typically, then, these studies are conducted with several participating centers and a coordinating center. Usually laboratory samples, images, and data are sent to the coordinating center, which carries out the data analysis and monitors the progress of the study to ensure that it follows the protocol and standard operating procedures. The larger number of patients included in this phase also provides a further opportunity for closely monitoring the safety of the drug. An independent data safety monitoring committee carefully follows the safety of the drug and may call for the termination of a trial if safety is inadequate or if the new treatment displays such great efficacy that it would be unethical for the patients on the control treatment to continue in the trial. Phase III trials are generally randomized, double-blind, controlled trials. Patients entering the trial are randomly assigned to either the new drug that is being tested (active treatment) or a control treatment. The control treatment may be a standard drug used in the treatment of a disease or a placebo, a fake treatment that appears convincingly like the active treatment under investigation. Double-blinding, also called double-masking, means that both the investigators performing assessments on the study subjects and the subjects being assessed in the trial do not know whether they are receiving the new treatment or the control treatment. In this way bias (factors that interfere with analyzing a trial) is minimized.

Phase IV: Postmarketing Surveillance

In Phase IV studies, the emphasis is on safety. When Phase III has been completed, the sponsor must file a new drug application with the FDA. The application involves voluminous documentation of the data on safety and efficacy that have been acquired across all phases of the study. FDA advisory committees, which are constituted to address specialized disease areas, recommend approval or disapproval of the drug. In addition to experts in the field, the committees include lay and patient representatives. Guidance documents are updated from time to time and are available at the FDA's Web site, www.fda.gov.

Here is a hypothetical example of the development of a new drug. It is known that cells called lymphocytes gather in salivary glands of Sjogren's patients as part of the immune and inflammatory process that fuels the disease. Dr. Sharp, a researcher at Clinical University, has discovered that biopsies of the salivary glands of her patients contain a unique type of lymphocyte that has not previously been described. It carries a distinctive molecule on its surface. She conducts studies in mice that have the same kind of inflammation in their glands, and finds that the animals also have lymphocytes with the distinctive surface molecule. She makes antibodies against the molecule to target these lymphocytes so that they can be destroyed, and finds that this dramatically diminishes the inflammation in the animals' salivary glands. Investigators at ABC Pharmaceuticals read her published report and are able to replicate her findings in the original mouse strain as well as another type of mouse with Sjogren's-like features. The company produces a humanized version of the antibody. The company investigates the immunological effects, toxicology, and dosing in several strains of animals with the mouse antibody as well as the new humanized antibody. In consultation with the FDA they perform further studies to establish the safety profile and then scale up production of pharmaceutical-grade antibodies for testing in humans. A protocol is written. The protocol is subject to scientific review to establish that the rationale and design of the study are sound. The documentation is sent to the IRBs of the institutions or groups that will participate in the trial. The major task of the IRBs is to ensure that the trial is ethical and safe and that the subjects will be adequately informed about what the study involves and its potential risks. New rules adopted in 2003 under the Health Insurance Portability and Accountability Act also apply to clinical trials which protect patients' confidentiality. The ABC pharmaceutical company then performs dosing and safety studies in healthy human subjects. If the drug successfully passes through Phases I through III, a new drug application can be filed with the FDA. If approved, production and marketing is undertaken and drug safety is further monitored in Phase IV postmarketing surveillance studies. After a decade of work and staggering costs, a new agent is available for the treatment of Sjogren's. (For existing drugs that have a well-known safety profile and are used for the treatment of related problems, testing for use in the treatment of Sjogren's is much less arduous.)

Marilyn Solsky, MD

Michael H. Weisman, MD

21 Adjunctive Measures, Comorbidities, and Reproductive Issues in Sjogren's

PATIENTS WITH SJOGREN'S SYNDROME are well aware of their symptoms of dry eye and dry mouth; however, Sjogren's is a systemic illness, and patients need to be aware of certain risk factors and comorbidities that exist with this disease. Patients with Sjogren's secondary to another rheumatic condition such as systemic lupus erythematosus (SLE) or rheumatoid arthritis (RA) need to be cognizant of the potential additional complications of these conditions.

Infections

Medications used to treat the chronic signs and symptoms of Sjogren's generally include at least one anti-inflammatory and often more. Nonsteroidal anti-inflammatory drugs (NSAIDs), corticosteroids, and immunosuppressants such as methotrexate or azathioprine all have the capability to suppress fevers. Any temperature a patient develops on these medications is extremely significant and should be immediately brought to the attention of a physician. The fever may represent an acute infection or a disease flare. Patients on immunosuppressants are susceptible to infections from organisms that usually do not affect those with intact immune systems; patients need to be aware that any acute change in symptoms, such as fatigue or malaise, may herald an infection, even if no temperature is present.

If a patient with Sjogren's is found to have an infection and is treated with an antibiotic, then there needs to be monitoring for the development of yeast infections. Sjogren's patients are especially prone to oral candidiasis because of decreased oral secretions. Many patients with autoimmune diseases are sulfa-sensitive, and if possible an alternative antibiotic should be used.

Allergies

Patients with allergies such as allergic rhinitis or hay fever often have elevated levels of an immunoglobulin called IgE. Levels of IgE are generally the same in patients with autoimmune diseases as in the general population. Patients with Sjogren's syndrome are no more prone to developing allergies than people without Sjogren's. However, the treatment for allergy symptoms often involves the use of a decongestant or antihistamine that can further exacerbate mouth and eye dryness. Fortunately, with some of the newer agents, such as cetirizine, fexofenadine, and loratadine, these sicca side effects have been minimized.

For allergy patients for whom symptomatic treatment is not helpful, allergy shots (called desensitization) are often recommended. However, patients with autoimmune diseases may react poorly to allergy shots, and the shots may cause disease flares. If allergy shots are indicated, then patients should proceed slowly, possibly with lower doses of the sensitizing allergen, and stop if there is a flare of the disease.

The best treatment for allergies, although it may not always be practical, is to avoid exposure to the allergen.

Osteoporosis

Patients with Sjogren's syndrome, and particularly patients with secondary Sjogren's, are at an increased risk for developing osteoporosis, especially if they are taking an anti-inflammatory medication such as methotrexate or corticosteroids. Corticosteroids affect bone mineralization almost immediately, and any patient on chronic steroids should be on an agent that treats osteoporosis. The American College of Rheumatology recommends obtaining a baseline bone density measurement for any patient receiving corticosteroids. All patients with chronic inflammatory diseases should be involved in a weight-bearing exercise program and should be taking 1,200–1,500 mg of calcium and 400 IU of vitamin D daily, unless they have a risk factor for developing kidney stones or have other kidney impairment.

Medications that are currently available for treating osteoporosis are calcitonin (by injection or nasal inhalation), the bisphosphonates, teriparatide, and selective estrogen receptor modulators. Teriparatide mimics the action of parathyroid hormone and stimulates the formation of new bone. The other agents inhibit further bone resorption. There are currently two oral bisphosphonates available, alendronate and risedronate; these are taken weekly on an empty stomach. Some patients may find that these medications cause severe esophagitis; for patients unable to take the oral bisphosphonates, the intravenous forms of the bisphosphonates, pamidronate or zolendronate, may be better tolerated. Teriparatide is an analogue of parathyroid hormone and is taken as a daily injection. Raloxifene is the most widely used estrogen receptor modulator; however, while it does help prevent osteoporosis and does not adversely affect breast tissue, it also does not prevent the problem of hot flashes.

Male patients with Sjogren's should have testosterone levels checked, since low testosterone levels are an additional risk factor for osteoporosis, and may be decreased in men with autoimmune diseases.

Autoantibodies, Neonatal Disease, and Pregnancy

Anti-Ro/SSA and Anti-La/SSB Antibodies

Antibodies are part of the body's normal defense mechanism; they usually are directed against foreign antigens such as bacteria, and will inactivate and destroy them. In autoimmune diseases, it is believed, there is a "misreading" of antigens and the antibodies become directed against the self's normal proteins, sometimes causing disease, rather than protecting against it. One of the criteria used for the diagnosis of Sjogren's syndrome is the presence of antibody to Ro/SSA and/or La/SSB. Different clinical associations have been identified with Ro/SSA or La/SSB, or both antigens together. Sometimes antibodies are merely markers of the presence of a disease and have little or no involvement in the pathogenesis or mechanisms that produce the disease. Anti-Ro/SSA has been associated with several clinical manifestations, including a low platelet count and a low white count in Sjogren's; it has also been associated with pulmonary disease in lupus. Both the anti-Ro/SSA and anti-La/SSB antibodies have been associated with development of congenital heart block in neonates and a syndrome referred to as neonatal lupus.

Pregnancy

During a healthy pregnancy the mother's antibodies are transported across the placenta into the bloodstream of the developing fetus. This movement of maternal antibodies across the placenta begins at or around the end of the first trimester. Because the fetus is incapable of making its own antibodies until after birth, these maternal antibodies are critical for helping the developing fetus fight infection. Unfortunately, the placenta cannot distinguish between antibodies that are beneficial for the fetus and those that may be harmful.

Mothers with Anti-Ro/SSA and Anti-La/SSB Antibodies

One of the most interesting associations of an antibody with clinical disease was the realization that anti-Ro/SSA and anti-La/SSB antibodies are associated with congenital heart block and a characteristic skin rash in neonates (see pages 76–77). This disease complex was termed neonatal lupus because the first babies who were noted to have heart block were born to women who had systemic lupus erythematosus. However, it is now understood that the pathology for these illnesses is not related to lupus but is conferred by the presence of the anti-Ro/SSA or anti-La/SSB antibody. At the time of the pregnancy the mother may not even be known to have SLE or Sjogren's. Whether or not a woman who has anti-Ro/SSA or anti-La/SSB antibody but is asymptomatic at the time of her pregnancy eventually develops a connective tissue disease is controversial. One long-term study has suggested that only about 2 percent of mothers who are asymptomatic during their pregnancy develop SLE. Other investigators feel that eventually all mothers with anti-Ro/SSA and anti-La/SSB antibodies will develop an autoimmune disease, although in one author's experience the disease occurred 26 years after the patient had delivered her baby. It appears that anti-Ro/SSA binds cardiac conduction tissue more strongly than other cardiac tissue. However, this does not completely explain the pathogenesis of the disease, because maternal cardiac conduction tissue is not adversely affected by the presence of this antibody. The conduction defect that the infants develop is quite serious and can lead to permanent heart block.

The rash the infants develop has a slightly raised texture but is generally flat and may be somewhat circular in appearance. The rash lasts as long as maternal immunoglobulin lasts in the newborn circulation, approximately six months.

Clinical testing for the presence of anti-Ro/SSA and anti-La/SSB antibodies can be done by one of two different testing methodologies, immunodiffusion or enzyme-linked immunosorbent assay (ELISA). Testing by immunodiffusion is less sensitive and may miss some lower levels of the antibody. The better test, and the one more widely used, is the ELISA, which tests a patient's blood against highly purified forms of the Ro/SSA and La/SSB antigens. The Ro/SSA antigen is composed of two separate proteins. The unit used for measuring the size of a protein is a kilodalton (kD). One of the Ro/SSA proteins is 52 kD, and the other is 60 kD. La/SSB is composed of one protein that is 48 kD in size. There is a test that can distinguish between the two sizes of Ro/SSA proteins, the immunoblot or Western blot. This distinction becomes relevant for women who have the anti-Ro/SSA antibody and wish to become pregnant.

Women who have the anti-Ro/SSA antibody who may be at lower risk for having infants with heart block have been demonstrated to have three characteristics: (1) they have low titers of anti-Ro/SSA antibodies, (2) they do not have anti-La/SSB antibodies, and (3) immunoblot shows antibodies only to the 60 kD anti-Ro/SSA antibody and not to the 52kD protein.

The overall occurrence of complete congenital heart block is 1 in every 20,000 births. Anti-Ro/SSA and/or anti-La/SSB was found in 83 percent of neonates with complete congenital heart block. If a mother has anti-Ro/SSA or anti-La/SSB antibodies, then the chances of her having an infant affected with neonatal lupus are between 1 and 5 percent. If she has already had a child with heart block, then the risk of having a second affected child may be as high as one in six. It is possible that if the first child had heart block, the second child will have a skin rash, or vice versa.

The rash that can occur with neonatal lupus is self-limiting and usually disappears by age eight months to one year. Of more concern is the risk of complete congenital heart block. A mother with the anti-Ro/SSA or anti-La/SSB antibody may not necessarily have any problems with her pregnancy. However, hers is considered a high-risk pregnancy and should be closely monitored. If this is her first pregnancy, then an echocardiogram should be obtained at about the 18th week of pregnancy and repeated at 6-week intervals until the 30th week. At about 30 weeks the infant's heart rate should be audible on routine obstetrical examination.

If a heart block is detected, it is unlikely to be reversible. Under these circumstances treatment is watchful waiting and following the infant with weekly echocardiograms. If the echocardiogram detects inflammation around the heart or if the heart block is not complete (referred to as second-degree heart block), then treatment with dexamethasone may be indicated.

If complete heart block is detected, then the infant may still be able to live a normal life even without a pacemaker, or the infant may require pacemaker placement within the first three months of life, or death may occur in utero. Based on the experience of Dr. Jill Buyon, who heads the National Institute of Arthritis and Musculoskeletal and Skin Diseases—funded research registry for neonatal lupus, of 113 infants with neonatal lupus, 19 percent died within the first three months and 58 percent required pacemakers.

Infants born with neonatal lupus do not appear to be at any increased risk for developing lupus in later life unless the mother has SLE. Any child born to a mother with SLE, especially if the child is a girl, has an approximately 10 percent increased risk for developing lupus.

Mothers Without Anti-Ro/SSA or Anti-La/SSB Antibodies

Women with primary Sjogren's syndrome who do not have antibodies to Ro/SSA or La/SSB do not have any additional risk factors for pregnancy. Women with Sjogren's syndrome secondary to another connective tissue disease, especially SLE, do have extra considerations for a high-risk pregnancy, but it is beyond the scope of this chapter to discuss these issues. Women with connective tissue diseases who are contemplating pregnancy are referred to their physicians for further information regarding special factors that may affect their pregnancy

Antiphospholipid Antibodies

Another antibody that may be present in patients with Sjogren's syndrome is the anticardiolipin antibody. This antibody is associated with certain hypercoaguable phenomenon that lead to clotting in the arteries and/or veins, and clinically may be present as phlebitis, blood clots to the lungs, occlusion of the blood vessels that provide circulation to the eye, heart attacks, small strokes, or recurrent spontaneous miscarriages. Anticardiolipin antibodies are part of a broader class of substances found in the blood, antiphospholipid antibodies. Sometimes these terms are used interchangeably, although they refer to slightly different compounds. Phospholipids are involved in blood clotting and constitute part of several different proteins that are associated with an increased risk for adverse clotting events. The first coagulation disorder described was identified in two patients with SLE. In laboratory testing the patients' blood appeared to be too thin because of the presence of a protein that interfered with blood clotting. But, in fact, this protein predisposed the patients to more clotting events, creating what is referred to as a hypercoaguable condition. It is now known that this protein is found in patients without lupus, but the initial name has remained, and the protein became known as the lupus anticoagulant. Subsequently several other phospholipid compounds that are associated with hypercoaguable states have been identified, most notably anti-beta-2-glycoprotein I. The clinical events associated with these antibodies have been referred to as the antiphospholipid antibody syndrome.

Mothers with Antiphospholipid Syndrome

Women who have the antiphospholipid antibodies, particularly antibodies to cardiolipin, are at greater risk for experiencing recurrent spontaneous abortions. Placental thrombosis results in frequent abortions in the first trimester and recurrent fetal loss in the second and third trimesters. Mothers with antiphospholipid antibodies may also experience significant lowering of their platelet counts (thrombocytopenia) during their pregnancy.

Besides having a role in spontaneous abortions, antiphospholipid antibodies have also been associated with preeclampsia, intrauterine growth retardation, and infertility.

The mere presence of the antiphospholipid antibody, however, does not automatically imply that any adverse event will occur. Different authors have reported varying experiences with patients who have antiphospholipid antibodies. In one author's experience, fewer than 31 percent of all patients with antiphospholipid antibodies ever experienced thrombosis. Other reports suggest that women with anticardiolipin antibodies will have a 50 to 75 percent chance of having fetal loss. The management of pregnant women with antiphospholipid antibody syndrome needs to be individually determined, based on whether this is a patient's first pregnancy, whether she has had other episodes of fetal wastage, or whether she has an active underlying connective tissue disease. Treatment usually includes low-dose aspirin therapy; in some cases heparin is used. Prednisone use is reserved for special circumstances. With anticoagulant therapy and careful monitoring, the chances of a normal term delivery is reported to be approximately 97 percent.

Immunizations

Patients with autoimmune diseases are more susceptible to infections, due either to the nature of the underlying illness or to the side effects of immunosuppressant medications. Although immunization against specific infections may provide additional protection, the use of some vaccinations must be avoided or approached with caution.

Immunization against influenza, pneumonia, and tetanus is generally safe but not always effective in patients on high doses of steroids or other immune suppressants. Unless there arise emergent reasons for administering these immunizations—for example, giving a tetanus vaccine after an acute puncture wound—these vaccines should probably be given only when patients are on a steroid dose of 20 mg a day or less, or when immune suppressants can be at least temporarily discontinued.

The smallpox vaccine should not be given to patients with Sjogren's syndrome or other connective tissue diseases because it is an attenuated live vaccine, and in patients who are immunosuppressed the vaccine can actually induce the disease. The safety of other live vaccines, such as polio, mumps, BCG, yellow fever, measles, or rubella, has not been established in patients who are on high doses of immunosuppressants. Patients who have children receiving these vaccines should avoid contact with their children's oral and fecal secretions for approximately two weeks.

For patients traveling to third world countries, the benefit of receiving immunization to hepatitis A or typhoid probably outweighs the risks, but it should be discussed with the patient's physician.

Meningococcal vaccines are directed against certain components of the bacterial capsule; most older children and young adults who receive the vaccine develop immunity. However, in a population of patients with no spleen who had been treated with chemotherapy and radiation therapy for a lymphoma, a poor antibody response was seen. The meningococcal vaccine appears to be safe for patients with connective tissue diseases but theoretically may not confer immunity to patients on high doses of immunosuppressants.

Lyme vaccine at present remains somewhat controversial, as there is theoretical concern that the vaccine could induce Lyme disease in genetically susceptible individuals. A decision to receive Lyme vaccine should be determined individually between patient and physician.

Since exacerbations of disease have been reported among SLE patients receiving hepatitis B vaccine, and the vaccine has also been thought to induce lupus, immunization against hepatitis B should be decided on an individual basis based on risk factors and in conjunction with the patient's physician.

The Comorbidities of Aging

Sjogren's syndrome tends to affect an older population; the mean age of patients who have Sjogren's syndrome is 55 years. In this age group, even persons not affected by Sjogren's may experience symptoms of mouth and eye dryness. The eye dryness may be aggravated by the use of contact lenses. In patients with Sjogren's syndrome these symptoms may be intensified by the use of medications used to treat conditions associated with aging, such as hypertension, muscle spasms, and urinary incontinence. Beta-blockers (alone or in combination with other drugs), propanolol, labetolol, alpha-blockers, and clonidine are antihypertension drugs that can cause increased dryness. Two medications used for treating muscle spasms, cyclobenzaprine and methocarbamol, are also associated with mouth dryness. This is also true for bethanechol and oxybutynin, used for treating incontinence. Over-the-counter preparations for relieving symptoms of congestion, including chlorpheniramine maleate, pseudoephedrine, and other medications combined with them, have the same side effect of dry mouth. Patient's with Sjogren's who take any of these drugs need to be aware that these medications can exacerbate their symptoms; if necessary, they should request that their physician place them on a different medication.

It has now been well established that patients with autoimmune diseases are at increased risk for cardiovascular complications, and this risk is greatly increased by the use of corticosteroids. One indicator for this risk factor is the level of homocysteine, a circulating protein in patients' blood that can be quantified by a simple laboratory test. Patients can find out from their physicians if their level of homocysteine is being monitored. Elevated levels, if found, can be lowered by taking folic acid.

Elevated blood pressure also occurs with an aging population. New data confirm that lower blood pressure readings (a systolic blood pressure of 120 or less and a diastolic blood pressure of 80 or less) are associated with a decreased incidence of heart disease and stroke. Patients need to be aware that NSAIDs and corticosteroids can elevate blood pressure, and they may need to take additional medications to keep their blood pressure within a normal range. Corticosteroids can also affect blood glucose levels and induce diabetes, which can cause further problems with hypertension and arteriosclerosis. A similar effect of steroids is seen on lipid levels. Elevations in cholesterol and triglycerides, seen in general in an older population, can be aggravated by the use of steroids.

Thyroid Disease

The most frequent organ-specific autoimmune disease in patients with Sjogren's syndrome is autoimmune thyroiditis. About half of patients with Sjogren's syndrome have thyroid disease. In a study of 77 patients with lupus, 8 patients who had thyroid disease also had Sjogren's syndrome. Sjogren's syndrome and autoimmune thyroid disease may be related to each other pathogenetically.

Gynecologic Considerations

Women with Sjogren's syndrome are often significantly bothered by vaginal dryness, painful intercourse, and vaginal yeast infections. If women do not discuss this problem with their physician, they may use petroleum jelly to help relieve their symptoms, and this actually results in more tissue injury, interferes with the vagina's natural cleansing mechanism, and can impair sperm mobility in couples trying to conceive. Cortisone creams are equally unhelpful, as they can further thin tissue and may promote yeast infections.

There are several preparations available (and some being developed) to help with this underreported but important symptom. Various sterile lubricants, including K-Y jelly, which is water soluble and not subject to the difficulties posed by petroleum jelly, and Surgilube are useful vaginal lubricants. Maxilube, Vagisil, Sylk, and Astroglide are also water-soluble and nonirritating but have different physical characteristics than K-Y and Surgilube. Two nonhormonal vaginal moisturizers that may be used to help with general vaginal dryness are Replens and Lubrin, which is a vaginal insert. A once-a-week vaginal lubricant, Vagikote, is undergoing clinical trials. Vagifem is an estrogen-based topical intravaginal preparation that when used twice weekly can help with atrophic vaginitis and vaginal dryness in postmenopausal women. Although the absorption of estrogen is much lower than with the use of an oral or transdermal estrogen preparation, there is still a risk associated with all estrogen preparations, and the use of estrogen replacement needs to be determined on an individual basis after discussion with a health professional.

Women with Sjogren's are at increased risk for yeast infections because of vaginal dryness. This risk is further increased by a compromised immune system and the use of corticosteroids, the use of antibiotics, and the loss of estrogen's protective effects on normal vaginal bacteria in postmenopausal women. Any diabetes or blood sugar abnormality also predisposes patients to vaginal yeast infections. The irritation of vaginal dryness may mimic symptoms of a vaginal yeast infection, and treatment should be given only after an accurate diagnosis has been established. Once a diagnosis is determined, effective treatment is available with over the counter preparations such as Gyne-Lotrimin. Vaginal creams may be more effective than vaginal suppositories because they provide more coverage. Fluconazole, a one-dose oral treatment, is more costly but more convenient for the treatment of vaginal yeast infections.

Summing Up

Beyond dry eye and dry mouth, patients with Sjogren's syndrome have several unique challenges, but by being aware of several treatable risk factors, such as osteoporosis, hypertension, and cardiovascular disease, and discussing therapeutic options regarding immunizations and symptomatic treatment with their physicians, patients with Sjogren's syndrome can decrease some of the comorbidities associated with this disease.

PART V

Outcomes and
Future Directions

What happens to Sjogren's patients? What can they look forward to? Fortunately, most individuals with the syndrome have a normal life expectancy. However, their quality of life often leaves a lot to be desired. Are there any new investigational approaches or promising leads? Where does our research stand? In this final section, potential breakthroughs are discussed within the context of discussing the natural course of the syndrome.

22 Can I Work?

SJOGREN'S SYNDROME is known to cause eye and mouth dryness, fatigue, fever, joint pain, and muscle pain, but it also involves organs such as the lung, kidney, brain, and lymph glands. The severity of the illness varies widely; it can even be life-threatening and result in disability and inability to work. The mean age of a patient with Sjogren's syndrome is around 55, which suggests that many of these patients may qualify for Medicare benefits and Social Security payments at age 65.

What Is Disability?

Disability can be defined in general terms as being unable to perform a task in the workplace because of signs or symptoms of an illness. The word *disability* has specific meaning in insurance policies, where it refers to a change in the patient's capacity to carry out specific personal, social, and job-related tasks due to the presence of impairment. An *impairment* is a physical or mental constraint resulting from an illness. Your physician determines this, though the presence of an impairment does not always mean that a patient is disabled. For example, the presence of swollen and tender joints on examination is an impairment and needs to be documented in the medical record. A *handicap* refers to the social consequences that result from having an impairment or disability. Examples of this is documentation of limitation of one or more life's activities that were previously normal for the patient, the use of an assistive device such as a wheelchair or prosthesis, or needing more time than necessary to complete a certain task.

Factors Contributing to Disease Severity in Determining Disability

There are various demographic and psychosocial factors that can combine with an ailment's signs and symptoms to determine whether the person becomes disabled or not, such as age, gender, personality, level of education, social support, and pressure from colleagues and family. Other factors that impact a person's ability to work include the type of work, whether the person is self-employed, and how experienced the person is in a specific line of work. All of these factors are important to consider in determining disability.

What State and Federal Programs Are Available to the Disabled Person?

The two major government programs that compensate a person for being unable to work include Social Security disability and workers' compensation. The Social Security Administration provides two programs, Social Security disability insurance (Title II) (SSDI, also called disability insurance benefits), and Supplemental Security Income (Title XVI) (SSI). Eligibility for federal and state medical insurance programs such as Medicare and Medicaid is contingent on qualifying for either SSDI or SSI.

Numerous private insurance companies also provide disability income provided the employer or patient pays a certain premium.

Social Security Disability Insurance (SSDI)

SSDI is a federally regulated program that was established in the 1950s under Title II of the Social Security Act. Employers and workers contribute to a trust fund in the form of deductions from their payroll taxes. Workers receive benefits based on lifetime contributions if they meet certain published criteria. SSDI is one of the largest disability insurance programs in the world.

In order to qualify for SSDI, the Social Security Administration requires the individual to be unable "to engage in any substantial gainful activity by reason of any medically determinable physical or mental impairment which can be expected to result in death or which has lasted or can be expected to last for a continuous period of not less than 12 months." Unlike some private insurance companies, SSDI does not provide partial disability compensation if the person is not able to work at his or her job but is able to work or be trained for another vocation even at the minimum wage. The program attempts to show some flexibility with the wide ranges of individual's impairments, education, and vocational achievements. An individual who has received SSDI for 24 months may qualify for Medicare.

Supplemental Security Income (SSI)

People who do not qualify for SSDI due to the lack of contributions to the Social Security program may qualify for SSI under Title XVI of the Social Security Act. This requires the estimation of the patient's financial assets by a means test. This program pays a monthly amount to financially strapped people who qualify for disability. Patients who qualify for SSI may also qualify for Medicaid, a state-sponsored medical insurance for people who are indigent and unable to work.

Workers' Compensation

Workers' compensation is a nationwide state-run mandatory program that has to be provided to all employees to cover them for on-the-job accidents or occupation-related illnesses. Most programs are privately owned or state-sponsored; there is also a federal program for federal employees through the Department of Labor. Any injury that occurs during work or an illness that can be proven to have resulted from or been exacerbated by their occupation is covered under this program regardless of any culpability on the part of the employee in its causation. Workers' compensation can pay claims for partial disability. As a result of the Americans with Disabilities Act, employers who have fifteen or more employees are mandated to modify the workplace to accommodate someone with a disability.

What Eligibility Criteria Are Necessary to Qualify for Social Security Disability?

A worker who is between 31 and 65 years of age who has contributed to Social Security for at least 20 out of the preceding 40 quarters may apply for SSDI. Unmarried minor children and spouses caring for minor or disabled children are also eligible. The Social Security Administration examines the medical and work history provided by the claimant for evidence that supports the inability of the employee to earn more than $700 per month and for objective assessment of the magnitude and degree of the impairment documented in the medical history.

How Does Social Security Determine if a Person Is Disabled?

First, the SSA determines if the individual can earn at least $700 per month. Next, objective signs confirming the validity of symptoms causing the impairment are looked at. These symptoms have to prevent the worker from carrying out his or her usual tasks. Finally, the impairment in question must meet the requirements set under the SSA list of defined impairments and levels of disease activity.

Social Security Administration List of Defined Impairments That Apply to Sjogren's Syndrome

Currently Sjogren's syndrome is not on the SSA's list of defined impairments. Disability for Sjogren's syndrome is currently applied under "Impairments of the Immune System" (section 14.00) using either the category "Systemic Lupus Erythematosus" or "Undifferentiated Connective Tissue Disease." The Sjogren's Syndrome Foundation has recently petitioned the commissioner for the SSA to include Sjogren's syndrome separately under the list of impairments in the immune system category. Further, they have suggested changes in the listing of impairments in the various organ systems that are affected by Sjogren's syndrome. For example, under "Special Senses" (section 2.00), the dryness and inflammation of the eyes specific to Sjogren's, and the disability it creates, would be listed if they were approved by the Social Security Administration. The various impairments that may apply to Sjogren's syndrome for disability are listed in Table 22.1.

What Happens if the Applicant's Impairment Does Not Meet the Listed Criteria?

A physician or a specially trained vocational specialist employed by the Social Security Disability Determination Service performs a physical abilities test if the person does not meet the listed criteria. The testing for specific abilities such as standing, sitting, lifting, carrying, pushing, pulling, and so on is called determination of the person's residual functional capacity. These abilities are measured against set Department of

TABLE 22.1 SOCIAL SECURITY DISABILITY IMPAIRMENTS POTENTIALLY APPLICABLE TO SJOGREN'S SYNDROME

1.00 *Impairment of the Musculoskeletal System*

Five types of impairments can be listed under this category:
  A. Loss of function in a limb or part of the body
  B. Disorders of the spine
  C. Postsurgical residual disability for at least 6 months
  D. Major joint damage, such as to the hip, knee, ankle, shoulder, elbow, wrist, or hand
  E. Decreased joint range of motion
Under this category, the following are included:
  1.02 Active inflammatory arthritis present on exam for at least 3 months in spite of active treatment and expected to continue for at least 12 months (must be corroborated by specific immunologic tests or test supporting the presence of inflammation)
  1.03 Arthritis of a major weight-bearing joint from any cause
  1.04 Arthritis of one major joint in each of the upper extremities
  1.05 Disorders of the spine such as a compression fracture

2.00 *Impairment of the Special Senses*

Two types of impairments may be applied to Sjogren's in special circumstances due to severe dry eye or inflammation of components of the eyeball. Hearing loss may be due to damage to the nerve that conducts sound to the brain or due to middle ear disease.
  A. Change in visual acuity, field of vision, muscle function, or a loss of visual efficiency
  B. A hearing impairment, vertigo (sensation of spinning), or loss of speech
Under this category, the following are included:
  2.03 Visual efficiency of the eye of 20 percent or less after correction (visual efficiency is the product of the percent of remaining visual acuity and the percent of remaining visual field efficiency)
  2.07 Severe disturbance of balance function

3.00 *Impairment of the Respiratory System*

Severe dryness of the airways can result in a chronic, debilitating cough. The following category of impairments may apply to Sjogren's syndrome:
  3.01 Chronic pulmonary insufficiency, defined as a decrease in the amount of air that can be ventilated out with maximal force and the lung capacity to enable oxygen to diffuse through the lung membranes (values obtained should be equal to or less than the minimum value on tables set up by the Social Security Administration)

continued

TABLE 22.1 *continued*

8.00 *Impairment of the Skin*

Extensive involvement of the skin that is not responsive to treatment and is expected to last at least 12 months may qualify for disability.

11.00 *Impairment of the brain and spinal cord*

Categories of impairments that may occur due to brain and spinal cord involvement due to Sjogren's include:

11.02 Epilepsy—seizures that occur more than once a month despite adherence to treatment for at least 3 months

11.04 Central nervous system accident—with persistent speech difficulty or comprehension or weakness in two limbs that impairs gait or function

11.14 Peripheral neuropathy—numbness or weakness of the hands or feet that impairs gait or function

12.00 *Impairment of mental function*

12.02 Organic mental disorders (psychological or behavioral abnormalities can result from brain or spinal cord involvement due to Sjogren's syndrome; testing must document loss of specific cognitive abilities and difficulty with activities of daily living or work)

13.00 *Neoplastic diseases (cancers)*

13.06 Lymph nodes—lymphoma with progressive disease that is not controlled with treatment (lymphoma may affect 5 to 7 percent of Sjogren's patients during the course of the illness; the risk for lymphoma is estimated to be 44 times greater than in the general population)

14.00 *Impairment of the immune system*

14.02 Systemic lupus erythematosus—this illness is characterized by fever, constitutional symptoms and multisystem involvement, usually fulfilling the 1982 Revised Criteria for the Classification of Systemic Lupus Erythematosus (Sjogren's syndrome is often listed under this category since a separate category does not exist)

14.03 Vasculitis—inflammation of the blood vessels due to infectious, allergic, or autoimmune causes (may occur due to connective-tissue disorders such as Sjogren's syndrome)

14.06 Undifferentiated connective tissue disorder—with major joint involvement or severe impairment of eye, lung, skin, or brain as defined under 1.00, 2.00, 3.00, 8.00, 11.00, 12.00 or 13.00

Labor standards and are used to determine whether the individual is capable of performing sedentary, light, medium, heavy, or very heavy work. The physical requirements for these various categories include:

TABLE 22.2

Type of work	Sitting	Standing	Lifting	Physical demands
Sedentary	Most of time	Occasional	Occasional ≤ 10 lbs	Very little
Light work	Half the time	Frequent	20 lbs max., frequent ≤ 10 lbs	Push or pull arm/ leg controls
Medium work	Part of time		Very often 50 lbs max., frequent ≤ 25 lbs	More strenuous than light work
Heavy work	Part of time		Very often 100 lbs max., frequent ≤ 50 lbs	More strenuous than medium work
Very heavy work	Part of time		≥ 100 lbs, frequent ≥ 50 lbs	More strenuous than heavy work

Other factors determining the residual functional capacity includes the ability for the person to hear and speak, and his or her mental faculties. The degree of fatigue suffered helps to determine this capacity as well. The examiner also determines how well the applicant carries out activities of daily living: grooming and hygiene, and social and locomotor functions. If the examiner determines that the person is not able to perform the activities of his or her job adequately based the applicant's age, training, education, and previous work experience, then the individual may be granted disability even if he or she does not meet the listed criteria.

Can Someone Petition to Have the Application Reexamined if It Has Been Rejected?

Most of the initial applications that are reviewed by the initial physician panel are rejected. A person may request to have another physician panel examine the case, at which point approximately a third of the applications are approved. Rejected applications may be filed in front of an administrative law judge; approximately 50 percent of these are approved. Petitions denied after this stage may be appealed to the Social

Security Council and ultimately to a U.S. district court. About 50 percent of all applications to the SSA are ultimately approved.

Are All Applicants Eligible for Vocational Rehabilitation?

All applicants are eligible for vocational rehabilitation if the SSA examiner feels that the person is capable of retraining in a different field. The disability payments are continued, and tuition and transportation fees for rehab are usually paid by the participating agencies. Vocational rehabilitation is a benefit offered by the Federal Rehabilitation Act of 1973. All states are required to have a vocational rehabilitation program, which is funded by both the federal and state governments. The program provides counselors who can evaluate the disabled person's ability and interest in different areas of work. They also provide living and schooling expenses, costs of job training, and special equipment purchasing, and assist in job placement. Usually the program covers most of the expenses of tuition and retraining, particularly for individuals who are indigent.

Can an Individual Work While Receiving Benefits?

The disability benefits continue for nine months while a person works and earns at least $200 a month. If the person has worked for a cumulative period of nine months, then the disability payments continue for a period of three months and then stop. The payments get reinstated for any month in the next three years if the applicant is not able to earn at least $700 a month during this period. Medicare benefits continue for at least 39 months even though the person has come off disability.

Summing Up

Most patients with Sjogren's syndrome are able to work and lead productive lives. However, a subset with more severe systemic disease or a malignancy have severe impairments that make them eligible for disability payments. Most Sjogren's patients can benefit from modifications in their work environment so that extremes of temperature and exposure to fumes and solvents are avoided and their workstations are modified to be ergonomic to help prevent and diminish disabling symptoms due to joint pain and fatigue or dry and painful eyes.

Clio P. Mavragani, MD

Stuart S. Kassan, MD

Haralampos M. Moutsopoulos, MD

23 What Will Happen To Me?

SJOGREN'S SYNDROME is a chronic disease without a cure. It's a tough disease to live with day in and day out. However, many tools are available to Sjogren's patients to help them live a long and productive life, as we have seen in previous chapters. No one can tell a patient what will happen to her or him over time, but we can talk about some of the potential complications. Sjogren's is said to be a "lifestyle-threatening" but not life-threatening disease. In fact, although the symptoms of Sjogren's syndrome, such as dry mouth and eyes, can negatively impact quality of life and are long-lasting, this disorder rarely completely incapacitates or shortens life span. In cases of secondary Sjogren's syndrome, outcome is related to the underlying disorder. Complications from primary Sjogren's syndrome can occur at various levels, depending on the organs involved.

Most of the patients with Sjogren's syndrome will have a mild, although sometimes debilitating, clinical course with no significant impact on their general health. Evidence from recent studies supports this view, showing that these patients live as long as their peers.

Late Sequelae: Extraglandular Complications and Lymphoma Development

One should not forget that a few patients suffer from severe Sjogren's syndrome, which can lead to the development of vasculitis and lymphoma in later life. The severe form of the disease usually presents with red spots on the lower legs (purpura), low complement (C4) levels, and cryoglobulins in the blood. Purpuric lesions can be itchy, do not blanch with pressure, and usually come and go. Complement is a protein that participates in our defense against microbes, while cryoglobulins are a special group of immunoglobulins that precipitate under cold temperatures.

Years after the diagnosis of the disease is established, these patients develop vasculitis, which is eventually associated with destruction of the blood vessel wall due to deposition of immune complexes (clusters of antibodies with their antigens). As a result, complement is activated. This is the reason why low levels of it are found in the blood. Two types of vessels are involved in vasculitis in patients with Sjogren's syndrome: small and medium-sized arteries. Involvement of small vessels leads to the development of purpura. When the small arteries of the peripheral nerves are affected, weakness or a sensation of numbness and/or pins and needles can occur in the hands and legs in a stocking/glove distribution. When the small vessels of the kidney are involved, glomerulonephritis can develop, manifested by the presence of blood in the urine (microscopic hematuria). On the other hand, when medium-sized vessels are affected, infarction and necrosis of the small bowel can occur. Anemia and a reduced number of lymphocytes (lymphopenia) are also noted in this group of patients.

Low complement levels have been found to be the strongest predictor for subsequent death in this patient group. At any given age the risk of death in this group of patients is twice as high as in the general population. In contrast, in the absence of purpura, low complement (C4) levels, and cryoglobulins in the blood, the disease course is benign and mortality rates are similar to those observed in the general population. It is important to note that in most of the cases, the severe features of the disease are found at the onset, when the diagnosis is made. Therefore, the doctor knows from the beginning that certain high-risk patients should be carefully evaluated at regular intervals.

Lymphomas are tumors of the lymphatic system. This system is a network of organs, ducts, and nodes that interact with the blood's circulatory system to transport a watery clear fluid called lymph throughout the body. The lymphatic system is also involved in the production and transport of lymphocytes, which are white blood cells that participate in the body's defense against foreign invaders.

The first, most common sign of lymphomas may be painless enlargement of one or more lymph nodes, usually in the neck, armpits, or groin. They can also cause systemic symptoms, referred to as B symptoms, that include drenching night sweats and weight loss. Fever is often present, which may occur only at night in episodes that last several days followed by periods of no fever. Patients with B symptoms usually have more extensive and severe disease.

Diagnosis of lymphoma is based on lymph node biopsy. A small piece of lymph node is removed and examined under the microscope. This is done generally under local anesthesia; however, sometimes, general anesthesia is required.

Two major types of lymphoma are recognized, depending on the histological findings on lymph node biopsy. These are referred to as Hodgkin's and non-Hodgkin's lymphomas. According to histological appearance and the type of cells that are present, these are also distinguished by grade, low or high.

It is of note that the prevalence of lymphoma in patients with Sjogren's syndrome is estimated to be approximately 4 percent. Lymphomas in Sjogren's syndrome are mainly low-grade non-Hodgkin's lymphomas, which arise frequently in the lymphoid tissues found in various mucosal sites of the body; they are called mucosa-associated lymphoid tissue (MALT) lymphomas. They tend to be localized mainly in the salivary glands, but they commonly involve other sites of the body such as lymph nodes, the nasopharynx, the lung, and the stomach. Bone marrow is rarely affected. B symptoms are not frequently reported. Median survival for these patients is approximately six years. However, a smaller percentage of patients develop more aggressive, high-grade lymphomas. Unfortunately, for these patients the median survival is approximately two years from the time of diagnosis.

Treatment of lymphomas in patients with Sjogren's syndrome is based on their histological grade. In low-grade localized lymphomas affecting the exocrine glands, a wait-and-watch policy is recommended, because in these patients the survival rate did not differ between treated and untreated patients. In low-grade disseminated lymphomas, a single chemotherapeutic agent is suggested. However, in patients with high-grade lymphomas or low-grade lymphomas transforming to high-grade, combination chemotherapy is required. Unfortunately, despite therapy, the

---

TABLE 23.1 PROGNOSTIC CONSIDERATIONS IN SJOGREN'S

- Two major types of complications of Sjogren's syndrome are recognized: glandular (exocrine glands) and extraglandular (systemic).
- Glandular complications include dental caries and mouth infections, opacification of the cornea with blurring of the vision, dry and brittle skin, painful sexual intercourse, difficulty in swallowing, and megaloblastic anemia.
- Extraglandular complications include kidney, lung, and liver involvement without severe sequelae in the majority of cases.
- Patients without systemic manifestations at the time of diagnosis (arthritis, Raynaud's phenomenon, dry cough, kidney and liver problems) are unlikely to develop such symptoms in the future.
- The presence of purpura, low complement levels, and cryoglobulins are adverse predictors for lymphoma development.
- Life expectancy in the majority of patients with Sjogren's syndrome is normal.

---

outcome in these patients is poor. Currently, we are not aware of predictive factors for development of high-grade lymphoma or for the transformation from low-grade to high-grade lymphoma.

In a recent study, the main causes of death for 11 out of 261 patients with Sjogren's syndrome who were followed for many years were reported. These included lymphoma, cardiac failure due to damage of the muscle of the heart, tumor of the parotid gland, inflammation of the blood vessels, emphysema (chronic lung disease characterized by obstruction of the bronchi), stroke, old age, and pulmonary embolism. The last of these is due to increased levels of gamma globulins, which lead to an increased tendency for clotting and plugging of the pulmonary vessels, manifested as shortness of breath and pain in the chest.

Summing Up

In conclusion, the overwhelming majority of Sjogren's syndrome patients have a generally mild course with a normal life expectancy. However, in the presence of negative predictors, the development of lymphoproliferative disorder is a possibility. In these cases, careful monitoring should be performed with regular follow-ups, in order to early detect and manage such a complication (see Table 23.1).

24 Is There Hope for a Cure?

WHAT CAN PATIENTS WITH SJOGREN's look forward to in the next decade or two? Advances in basic medical science, especially immunology, genetics, and pharmacology, certainly offer hope that Sjogren's can be conquered, if not cured. This chapter will review some of the most promising current areas of investigation, but the cure may come from research as yet unknown.

Basic research that could lead to a cure for Sjogren's syndrome falls into two main categories. One category relates to the underlying immunologic mechanisms that lead to autoimmune diseases in general and to Sjogren's in particular. The other relates to the mechanisms of water transport across cell membranes and the hormones and other mediators that control the process.

As described in Chapter 5, autoimmunity reflects an immune system that is out of control. A simple, general scheme for this process might include environmental factors and a breakdown in a normal barrier such that a self-protein or antigen is strongly presented to an immune system with a genetic predisposition to respond in a way that perpetuates the response, leading to chronic inflammation and tissue damage. Inflammatory bowel disease (IBD) might illustrate this process. It is thought that the combination of a breakdown in the integrity of the lining of the small intestine and a change in the bacteria that inhabit the intestines leads to the presentation of a new antigen or antigens to the lymphocytes that are always abundant beneath the intestinal lining. This initiates a local immune and inflammatory response that in some predisposed individuals continues as a chronic process. The antigen in IBD is unknown, and there are likely to be many possible antigens. The antigens in some other autoimmune diseases, such as type 1 diabetes, are known; in Sjogren's, several candidates—such as the muscarinic M3 receptors and the recently described protein ICA69 (Chapter 4), which are present in salivary glands—may play a role.

Even if the process leading to autoimmunity in Sjogren's and other diseases is completely understood, it may be quite a while before this knowledge is translated into effective treatment or a cure. In the meantime, two more immediate, if less disease-specific, approaches are being actively explored. The first is to transplant organs or glands. Advances in chemotherapy to prevent rejection and more exciting methods to induce tolerance of transplanted tissue hold promise in the transplantation of the pancreatic islets, which produce insulin in patients with type 1 diabetes. Similar experiments are under way to transplant salivary glands in mice as a first step to develop this approach to the treatment of Sjogren's. A related approach is to use the same methods to induce tolerance to the offending antigens, as described above.

A second exciting area of basic research related to Sjogren's deals with aquaporins, the molecules that actually move water across the cell membranes of glands and into the ducts, which eventually leads to saliva in the mouth and tears in the eye. The movement of water is an active process that appears to be under positive and negative control by mediators such as the autonomic nervous system, acetylcholine, and nitric oxide. Detailed knowledge of the mechanisms of water transport and its control can lead to the development of pharmacologic agents to increase the flow of saliva and tears, but these agents would act only upon glands that were not yet destroyed and maintained some residual glandular function. This approach would not technically represent a cure, since such pharmacologic agents would do nothing to stop the underlying immune process and the continuing inflammation and destruction of the glands (see Table 24.1).

Under a mandate from Congress, the National Institutes of Health has established an Autoimmune Diseases Coordinating Committee, which in turn has produced an Autoimmune Diseases Research Plan. As this plan gets implemented by the various components of NIH and there

TABLE 24.1 CURRENT RESEARCH STRATEGIES FOR NEW TREATMENTS IN SJOGREN'S SYNDROME

Improved drugs to control inflammation
    Nonsteroidal anti-inflammatory agents (e.g., COX-3 inhibitors)
    Improved antimalarials (e.g., pure isomers)
    Improved corticosteroids (e.g., budesonide derivatives)
    Improved immunosuppressives
    Newer anticytokine agents
Improved drugs to treat dryness
    Autonomic-system-mediated therapies
    Neurotransmitter-mediated therapies
    New delivery systems (e.g., aquaporins)
Biologic agents for Sjogren's
    Targeting M3 receptors
    Tolerizing agents (e.g., peptides, vaccines)
Gene therapies
    Transplantation of salivary glands
    Measures to prevent lymphoma

is increased support for research on the individual autoimmune diseases, including Sjogren's (which has a prominent place in the research plan), patients with Sjogren's can look forward to ever more targeted research on Sjogren's and with it the hope for a cure.

PART VI

Appendices

APPENDIX 1
FOR FURTHER READING

Chapter 1—The History of Sjogren's Syndrome

Wollheim FA, A humble gentleman at 100, Clin Exp Rheumatol 1999; 17: 648–652.

Morgan WS, Castleman B, A clinicopathologic study of "Mikulicz's disease," Amer J Pathol 1953; 29: 471–503.

Bloch KJ, Buchanan WW, Wohl MJ, Bunim JJ, Sjogren's syndrome: a clinical, pathological and serological study of 62 cases, Medicine 1965; 44: 187–231.

Chapter 2—What Is Sjogren's Syndrome?

Bloch KJ, Buchanan WW, Wohl MJ, Bunim JJ, Sjogren's syndrome. a clinical, pathological and serological study of 62 cases, Medicine 1965; 44: 187–231.

Vitali C, Bombardiere S, Jonsson R, Moutsopoulos HM, Alexander EL, Carson SE, Daniels TE, Fox PC, Fox RI, Kassan SS, Pillemer SR, Talal N, Weissman MH, Classification criteria for Sjogren's syndrome: a revised version of the European Criteria proposed by the American European group. Ann Rheum Dis 2002; 61: 554–558.

Chapter 3—Who Develops Sjogren's Syndrome?

Garcia-Carrasco M, Ramos-Casals M, Rosas J, Pallares L, Calvi-Alen J, Cervera R, Font J, Ingelmo M, Primary Sjogren's syndrome: clinical and immunologic disease patterns in a cohort of 400 patients, Medicine (Baltimore) 2002; 81: 270–280.

Pillemer SR, Matteson EL, Jacobsson LT, Martens PB, Melton LJ, O'Fallon WM, Fox PC, Incidence of physician-diagnosed primary Sjogren's syndrome in residents of Olmstead County, Minnesota, Mayo Clin Proc 2001; 76: 593–599.

225

Thomas E, Hay EM, Hajeer A, Silman AJ, Sjogren's syndrome: a community-based study of prevalence and impact, Br J Rheumatol 1998; 37: 685–686.

Chapter 4—What Leads to Dryness?

Pflugfelder, SC, Solomon A, Stern ME, The diagnosis and management of dry eye: a twenty-five-year review. Cornea 2000; 19(5): 644–649.

Fox RI, Sjogren's syndrome: current therapies remain inadequate for a common disease. Exp Opin Invest Drugs 2000; 9(9): 2007–2016.

Atkinson JC, Fox PC, Sjogren's syndrome: oral and dental considerations. J Am Dent Assoc 1993 Mar; 124(3): 74–76, 78–82, 84–86.

Chapter 5—Sjogren's Syndrome: A Genetic and Immunologic Perspective

James JA, Harley JB, Scofield RH, Role of viruses in systemic lupus erythematosus and Sjogren's syndrome, Curr Opin Rheumatol 2000; 13: 370–376.

Vitali C, Bombardiere S, Jonsson R, Classification criteria for Sjogren's syndrome: a revised version of the European criteria proposed by the American-European Consensus Group, Ann Rheum Dis 2002; 61: 554–558.

Daniels TE, Sjogren's syndrome: clinical spectrum and current diagnostic controversies. Adv Dent Res 1996; 10: 3–8.

Manoussakis MN, Moutsopoulos HM, Sjogren's syndrome: current concepts, Adv Intern Med 2001; 47: 191–217.

Chapter 6—Generalized Symptoms and Signs of Sjogren's Syndrome

Tziofas AG, Moutsopoulos H, Sjogren's syndrome, in *Rheumatology*, 3rd edition, MC Hochberg et al., eds., Mosby, 2003, pp. 1431–1443.

Pavlidis NA, Karsh J, Moutsopoulos HM, The clinical picture of primary Sjogren's syndrome: a retrospective study, J Rheumatol 1982; 9: 685–690.

Klippel J, Dieppe P, eds., *Rheumatology*, 2nd edition, Mosby, 1998.

Kelley W, Harris E, Ruddy S, Sledge C, *Textbook of rheumatology*, 4th edition, Saunders, 1993.

Carsons S, Daniels T, Dana R, Talal N, Sjogren's syndrome: new insights and new treatment, Winthrop University Hospital, 2001.

Carsons S ed., *The new Sjogren's syndrome handbook*, Oxford University Press, 1998.

Chapter 7—The Dry Eye

Lemp MA, Report of the National Eye Institute/Industry workshop on clinical trials in dry eyes, CLAO J 1995; 21: 221–232.

Dana, MR, Hamrah P, Role of immunity and inflammation in corneal and ocular surface disease associated with dry eye, Adv Exp Med Biol 2002; 506: 729–738.

Argueso P, Balaram M, Spurr-Michaud S, Keutmann HT, Dana MR, Gipson IK, Decreased levels of the goblet cell mucin MUC5AC in tears of patients with Sjogren syndrome, Invest Ophthalmol Vis Sci 2002; 43: 1004–1011.

Chapter 8—The Salivary Glands, Ears, Nose, and Larynx

Sharp K, Sjogren's syndrome, Gale Encyclopedia of Alternative Medicine, K Krapp and JL Longe eds., Gale, 2001.

Martin D, Sjogren's syndrome, Johns Hopkins Arthritis Center.

National Oral Health Information Clearinghouse, Dry mouth brochure, 1 NOHIC Way, Bethesda, MD.

Chapter 9—The Dry Mouth: A Dental Perspective on Sjogren's

Navazesh M, How can oral health care providers determine if patients have dry mouth? JADA 2003; 134: 613–620.

Daniels TE, Wu AJ, Xerostomia—clinical evaluation and treatment in general practice, CDA Journal 2000; 28: 933–941, available at http://www.cda.org/member/pubs/journal/jour1200/xero.html.

Mandel I, Surattanont F, Bilateral parotid swelling: a review, Oral Surg Oral Med Oral Pathol Oral Radiol Endod 2002; 93: 221–237.

Chapter 10—The Internal Organs in Sjogren's

Tzioufas AG, Moutsopoulos HM, Sjogren's syndrome, in *Rheumatology*, 2nd edition, J Klippel and P Dieppe eds., Gower, 1998, 32.1–12.

Manoussakis MN, Moutsopoulos HM, Sjogren's syndrome: current concepts, Advances in Internal Medicine 2001; 47: 191–217.

Soliotis FC, Mavragani CP, Moutsopoulos HM, Central nervous system involvement in Sjogren's syndrome, Annals Rheum Dis 2004; 63: 616–620.

Kassan, SS, Moutsopoulos, HM, Clinical manifestations and early diagnosis of Sjogren's Syndrome, Arch Intern Med, 164: 1275–1284, 2004.

Chapter 11—Manifestations of Connective Tissue Diseases Seen in Secondary Sjogren's

Klippel J, Crofford L, Stone J, Weyand C eds., *Primer on the Rheumatic Diseases*, Arthritis Foundation, 2001.

Kelley W, Harris E, Ruddy S, Sledge C eds., *Textbook of Rheumatology*, Saunders, 1997.

Wallace D, Hahn B eds., Dubois' Lupus Erythematosus, Lippincott Williams and Wilkins, 2002.

Chapter 12—Useful Studies: Blood Tests, Imaging, Biopsies, and Beyond

Garcia-Carrasco M, Ramos-Casals M, Rosas J, Pallares L, Calvo-Alen J, Cervera R, Primary Sjogren's syndrome: clinical and immunologic disease patterns in a cohort of 400 patients, Medicine 2002; 81: 270–280.

Vitali C, Bombardiere S, Jonsson R, Moutsopoulos HM, Alexander EL, Carson SE, Daniels TE, Fox PC, Fox RI, Kassan SS, Pillemar SR, Talal N, Weissman MH, Classification criteria for Sjogren's syndrome: a revised version of the European Criteria proposed by the American European group, Ann Rheum Dis 2002; 61: 554–558.

Markusse HM, Pillay M, Breedveld FC, The diagnostic value of salivary gland scintigraphy in patients suspected of primary Sjogren's syndrome, Br J Rheum 1993; 32: 231–235.

Chapter 13—How Can I Be Sure It's Really Sjogren's?

Schein, OD, Hochberg, MC, Munoz B, et al., Dry eye and dry mouth in the elderly: a population-based assessment. Arch Int Med. 1999; 159: 1359.

Itescu S, Winchester R, Diffuse infiltrative lymphocytosis syndrome: a disorder occurring in human immunodeficiency virus-1 infection that may present as a sicca syndrome, Rheumatic Diseases Clinics of North America 1992; 18(3): 683–697.

Loustajud-Ratti V, Riche A, Liozon E, Labrousse F, Soria P, Rogez S, Babany G, Delaire L, Denis F, Vidal E, Prevalence and characteristics of Sjogren's syndrome or sicca syndrome in chronic hepatitis C virus infection: a prospective study, Journal of Rheumatology 2001; 10: 2245–2251.

Chapter 14—Treatment of Dry Eye

Bron AD, Diagnosis of dry eye, Surv Ophthalmol 2001; 45 supp. 2: S221–226.

Pflugfelder SC, Solomon A, Stein ME, The diagnosis and management of dry eye, Cornea 2000; 19: 644–649.

Schaumberg DA, Buring JE, Sullivan DA, Dana MR, Hormone replacement therapy and dry eye syndrome, JAMA 2001; 286: 2114–2119.

Chapter 15—Treatment of Dry Mouth

Al-Hashimi I, The management of Sjogren's syndrome in dental practice, J Am Dent Assoc 2001; 132: 1409–1417.

Brennan MT, Shariff G, Lockhart PB, Fox PC, Treatment of xerostomia: a systematic review of therapeutic trials, Dent Clin N Am. 2002; 46: 847–856.

Grisius MM, Salivary gland dysfunction: a review of systemic therapies, Oral Surg Oral Med Oral Pathol 2001; 92: 156–162.

Chapter 16—Systemic Therapies in Sjogren's

Linardaki G, Moutsopoulos HM, The uncertain role of immunosuppressive agents in Sjogren's syndrome, Cleve Clin J Med 1997; 64: 523–526.

Moutsopoulos NM, Moutsopoulos HM, Therapy of Sjogren's syndrome, Springer Semin Immunopathol 2001; 23: 131–145.

Tzioufas AG, Moutsopoulos HM, Sjogren's syndrome, in *Rheumatology*, 3rd edition, J Smolen et al. eds., Gower, 2003.

Chapter 17—Taming Sjogren's: Fighting Fatigue, Lifestyle Factors, and Nondrug Management

Melvin J, Fibromyalgia—Getting Healthy, American Occupational Therapy Association, Rockville, MD, 1996.

Chapter 18—Conquering Sjogren's

Barendregt PJ, Visser MR, Smets EM, Tulen JH, van den Meiracker A, Boomsma F, Markusse HM, Fatigue in primary Sjogren's syndrome, Ann Rheum Dis 1998; 57: 291–295.

Broderick JE, Mind-body medicine in rheumatologic disease, Rheumatic Disease Clinics of North America 2000; 26: 161–176.

Rumpf TP, Hammitt KM, *The Sjogren's Syndrome Survival Guide*, New Harbinger, 2003.

Valtysdottir ST, Gudbjornsson B, Lindqvist U, Hallgren R, Hetta J, Anxiety and depression in patients with primary Sjogren's syndrome, J Rheumatol 2000; 27: 165–169.

Chapter 19—Complementary and Alternative Therapies for Sjogren's

Complementary and Alternative Therapies for Rheumatic Conditions, Rheumatic Disease Clinics of North America 1999; 25(4), and 2000; 26(1) 2000.

Lad VD, *Ayurveda: the science of self-healing*, 2nd edition, Lotus, 1985.

Rotblatt M, Ziment I, Evidence-based herbal medicine, Hanley and Belfus, 2001.

Additional references cited can be obtained by contacting Dr. Venuturupalli directly.

Chapter 20—How Are Drugs Tested for Sjogren's?

1. Anaya JM, Talal N, Sjogren's syndrome comes of age. Semin Arthritis Rheum 1999; 28:355–9.

2. Vivino FB, Al-Hashimi I, Khan Z, et al., Pilocarpine tablets for the treatment of dry mouth and dry eye symptoms in patients with Sjogren syndrome: a randomized, placebo-controlled, fixed-dose, multicenter trial. P92-01 Study Group. Arch Intern Med 1999; 159:174–81.

3. Petrone D, Condemi JJ, Fife R, Gluck O, Cohen S, Dalgin P, A double-blind, randomized, placebo-controlled study of cevimeline in Sjogren's syndrome patients with xerostomia and keratoconjunctivitis sicca. Arthritis Rheum 2002; 46:748–54.

4. Vitali C, Bombardieri S, Jonsson R, et al., Classification criteria for Sjo-

gren's syndrome: a revised version of the European criteria proposed by the American-European Consensus Group. Ann Rheum Dis 2002; 61: 554–8.

5. Bowman SJ, Pillemer S, Jonsson R, et al., Revisiting Sjogren's syndrome in the new millennium: perspectives on assessment and outcome measures. Report of a workshop held on 23 March 2000 at Oxford, UK. Rheumatology (Oxford) 2001; 40:1180–8.

6. Kaitin KI, Bryant NR, Lasagna L, The role of the research-based pharmaceutical industry in medical progress in the United States. J Clin Pharmacol 1993; 33:412–7.

7. Anello C, Emerging and recurrent issues in drug development. Stat Med 1999; 18:2301–9.

8. Lipsky MS, Sharp LK, From idea to market: the drug approval process. J Am Board Fam Pract 2001; 14:362–7.

9. Kaitin KI, Melville A, Morris B, FDA advisory committees and the new drug approval process. J Clin Pharmacol 1989; 29:886–90.

10. Ellenberg SS, Independent data monitoring committees: rationale, operations and controversies. Stat Med 2001; 20:2573–83.

Chapter 21—Adjunctive Measures, Comorbidities, and Reproductive Issues in Sjogren's

Bick RL, Antiphospholipid thrombosis syndromes, Hematol Oncol North America 2003; 17(1): 115–147.

Buyon, JP, Pregnancy in women with Sjogren's syndrome: neonatal problems, in *The new Sjogren's syndrome handbook*, S Carsons, EK Harris eds., Oxford University Press, 1998, 134–139.

Fox RI, Michelson P, Tornwall J, Approaches to the treatment of Sjogren's syndrome, in *Textbook of Rheumatology*, S Ruddy, ED Harris Jr., CB Sledge eds., Saunders, 2001, 1027–1038.

Chapter 22—Can I Work?

Disability evaluation under social security, Social Security Administration, Office of Disability, 1999.

Chapter 23—What Will Happen to Me?

Ioannidis JP, Vassiliou VA, Moutsopoulos HM, Long-term risk of mortality and lymphoproliferative disease and predictive classification of primary Sjogren's syndrome, Arthritis Rheum. 2002; 46: 741–747.

Skopouli FN, Dafni U, Ioannidis JP, Moutsopoulos HM, Clinical evolution and morbidity and mortality of primary Sjogren's syndrome, Semin Arthritis Rheum 2000; 29: 296–304.

Voulgarelis M, Moutsopoulos HM, Lymphoproliferation in autoimmunity and Sjogren's syndrome, Curr Rheumatol Rep 2003; 5: 317–323.

Chapter 24—Is There Hope for a Cure?

Winer S et al., Primary Sjogren's syndrome and deficiency of ICA69, Lancet 2002; 360: 1063–1069.

Hakala M, Niemela R, Does autonomic impairment have a role in pathophysiology of Sjogren's syndrome? Lancet 2000; 355: 1032–1033.

APPENDIX 2
RESOURCE MATERIALS

Organizations

The Sjogren's Syndrome Foundation
Web site: www.sjogrens.org
Phone: 800-475-6473, 301–718-0300

The primary source of information and support for Sjogren's syndrome, specifically serving Sjogren's patients and health care providers. Offers a wealth of materials and information on Sjogren's syndrome, related symptoms, and overlapping disorders. Watch the SSF Web site for information on Sjogren's, resource materials, educational seminars, support group meetings, contacts, and research and advocacy initiatives in Sjogren's. You may also call 800-475-6473 or 301-718-0300 to speak with a foundation staff member. Join the foundation and receive the *Moisture Seekers* newsletter to stay informed about the newest treatments and research and learn about practical tips and strategies for coping with Sjogren's. Made up of top clinicians and researchers in Sjogren's from around the world, the SSF Medical and Scientific Advisory Board authors, reviews, and recommends materials, and serves as a clearinghouse for medical information on Sjogren's.

Your membership not only provides you with access to up-to-date information, but your membership and donations also support the work of the foundation as cited in its mission to:

- Educate patients and their families about Sjogren's syndrome
- Increase public and health care provider awareness of Sjogren's syndrome
- Encourage research for new treatments and a cure

Many resource materials are available from the Sjogren's Syndrome Foundation, including books, pamphlets, brochures, audiotapes, and educational as well as exercise videos. In addition, SSF maintains lists of treatment centers and products. Try the SSF and the SSF Store (found at www.sjogrens.org) first!

While the Sjogren's Syndrome Foundation provides information on related and overlapping diseases, you might also wish to contact other not-for-profit organizations that focus solely on these diseases or include Sjogren's syndrome in their education. These organizations include:

American Autoimmune Related Diseases Association
Web site:www.aarda.org
Phone: 586-776-3900

Arthritis Foundation
Web site:www.arthritis.org
Phone: 800-283-7800

Lupus Foundation of America, Inc.
Web site:www.lupus.org
Phone: 202-349-1155

Lupus Research Institute
Web site:www.lupusresearchinstitute.org
Phone: 212-685-4118

Scleroderma Foundation
Web site: www.scleroderma.org
Phone: 800-722-4673

Scleroderma Research Foundation
Web site: www.srfcure.org
Phone: 800-441-2873

Federal Government Resource and Treatment Center
Sjogren's Syndrome Clinic
National Institute of Dental and Craniofacial Research
Building 10, Room 1N113
10 Center Drive MSC 1190
Bethesda, MD 20892-1190
Phone: 301-435-8528
http://wwwdir.nidcr.nih.gov/dirweb/gttb/sjogrens/SjogrenIndex.asp

Books Specifically on Sjogren's Syndrome
The Sjogren's Syndrome Survival Guide, by Teri P. Rumpf, PhD, and Katherine Morland Hammitt, New Harbinger Publications, 2003
    This invaluable resource on Sjogren's syndrome provides the latest medical information, research results, and treatment methods available as well as effective self-help strategies. Patients learn how to improve their quality

of life by taking an active role in their care and developing true partnerships with their doctors. Hammitt compiles clear answers to questions she and many other Sjogren's patients long found inaccessible, while Rumpf, a clinical psychologist, covers aspects of relationships, work, and finding informed and supportive medical care.

A Body Out of Balance: Understanding and Treating Sjogren's Syndrome,
    by Ruth Fremes and Nancy Carteron, Avery/Penguin Putnam, 2003
    Fremes, a Sjogren's patient, discusses Sjogren's symptoms, while her doctor, Carteron, explains the biological process, diagnosis, and treatment. This book provides readers with a comprehensive guide to the wide array of symptoms of Sjogren's, traditional and complementary treatments, and coping mechanisms for patients to devise their own holistic personal treatment plan.

Understanding Sjogren's Syndrome, by Sue Dauphin, Pixel Press, 1993
    Dauphin's book is filled with practical advice and an easy-to-understand explanation of Sjogren's syndrome. She covers the seriousness of this disease with a wonderful sense of humor and examples from her own and other patients' experiences.

The Official Patient's Sourcebook on Sjogren's Syndrome: A Revised and
    Updated Director for the Internet Age, edited by James N. Parker and
    Philip M. Parker, ICON Group International, 2002
    In addition to providing basic information on Sjogren's syndrome, the authors explain how to search for and find practical information. Directions focus on Internet use and include instruction on finding information about clinical trials, research studies on Sjogren's, medications, alternative medicine, nutrition, medical libraries, and insurance rights.

Pamphlets Specifically on Sjogren's Syndrome

Products Used by People with Sjogren's Syndrome, published by the Sjogren's Syndrome Foundation and updated regularly
    This pamphlet lists prescription and over-the-counter drugs and products for common symptoms of Sjogren's, the company that produces each item, and how to contact those manufacturers. Copies are available from the Sjogren's Syndrome Foundation by calling 301-718-0300 or e-mailing ssf@sjogrens.org. SSF members can also download a copy from the Web site at www.sjogrens.org.

Sjogren's Syndrome Self-Help: Tips for More Comfortable Living, by Dona Frosio, introduction by Steven Taylor, published by the Sjogren's Syndrome Foundation, first published in 1996, and revised in 2001 and in 2003

This pamphlet was authored by a Sjogren's syndrome patient, foundation support group president, and frequent speaker at foundation meetings. Frosio offers helpful ideas for living with Sjogren's based on her own experiences and those contributed by others with Sjogren's. Copies are available from the Sjogren's Syndrome Foundation by calling 301-718-0300 or e-mailing ssf@sjogrens.org. SSF members can also download a copy from the Web site at www.sjogrens.org.

Questions and Answers about Sjogren's Syndrome, a publication of the U.S. Department of Health and Human Services, National Institutes of Health, National Institute of Arthritis and Musculoskeletal and Skin Diseases, 2001, NIH Publication No. 01-4861
The Sjogren's Syndrome Foundation assisted NIAMS in the compilation of this Q&A booklet, which includes answers to common questions about Sjogren's syndrome, including symptoms, causes, diagnosis, and treatment. Copies are available from NIAMS, NIH, 1 AMS Circle, Bethesda, MD 20892-3675, or on the NIAMS Web site at www.nih.gov/niams/healthinfo. It may be viewed online at www.niams.nih.gov/hi/topics/sjogrens/index.htm.

Dry Mouth (Xerostomia), a publication of the National Institutes of Health (NIH), National Institute of Dental and Craniofacial Research, 2002, NIH Publication No. 02-3174
This brochure discusses the causes of dry mouth, the importance of saliva to oral health, provides steps to follow to relieve dryness, and includes information on the Dry Mouth/Sjogren's Syndrome Clinic at the National Institute of Dental and Craniofacial Research. Copies are available by writing the National Oral Health Information Clearinghouse, 1 NOHIC Way, Bethesda, Maryland 20892-3500, or calling them at 301-402-7364. You can also order or download a copy from the NIH Web site at http://www.nohic.nidcr.nih.gov/cgi-bin/ohpubgen_new.

Highly Recommended Books on Coping with Chronic Illness
A Delicate Balance: Living Successfully with Chronic Illness, by Susan Milstrey Wells, Perseus Publishing, 1998
Finding the Way Home: A Compassionate Approach to Illness, by Gayle Heiss, QED Press, 1997
Beyond Chaos: One Man's Journey Alongside His Chronically Ill Wife, by Gregg Piburn, Arthritis Foundation, 1999
The Chronic Illness Workbook: Strategies and Solutions for Taking Back Your Life, by Patricia A. Fennell, New Harbinger Publications, 2001
Sick and Tired of Feeling Sick and Tired: Living with Invisible Chronic Illness, by Paul J. Donoghue and Mary E. Siegel, W. W. Norton, 2000

Practical Guides

Disability Workbook for Social Security Applicants, by Douglas M. Smith, Physicians' Disability Services, Inc., 5th edition, 2001

Arthritis Today Drug Guide, Arthritis Foundation, updated annually

Books on Related and Overlapping Diseases and Symptoms

The Autoimmune Connection: Essential Information for Women on Diagnosis, Treatment, and Getting On with Your Life, by Rita Baron-Faust and Jill P. Buyon, McGraw-Hill/Contemporary Books, 2003

Living Well with Autoimmune Disease: What Your Doctor Doesn't Tell You That You Need to Know, by Mary J. Shomon, HarperCollins, 2002

Thriving with Your Autoimmune Disorder: A Woman's Mind-Body Guide, by Simone Ravicz, New Harbinger, 2000

Numb Toes and Aching Soles: Coping with Peripheral Neuropathy, by John A. Senneff, MedPress, 1999

Numb Toes and Other Woes: More on Peripheral Neuropathy, by John A. Senneff, MedPress, 2001

The Lupus Book: A Guide for Patients and Their Families, by Daniel J. Wallace, Oxford University Press, 1995

Coping with Lupus, by Robert Phillips, Avery, 2001

Lupus: Everything You Need to Know, by Robert G. Lahita and Robert H. Phillips, Avery, 1998

All About Fibromyalgia: A Guide for Patients and Their Families, by Daniel J. Wallace and Janice Brock Wallace, Oxford University Press, 2002

The Interstitial Cystitis Survival Guide: Your Guide to the Latest Treatment Options and Coping Strategies, by Robert M. Moldwin, New Harbinger, 2000

Coping with Chronic Fatigue Syndrome: Nine Things You Can Do, by Fred Friedberg, New Harbinger, 1995

The Scleroderma Book: A Guide for Patients and Families, by Maureen D. Mayes, Oxford University Press, 1999

All About Osteoarthritis: The Definitive Resource for Arthritis Patients and Their Families, by Nancy E. Lane and Daniel J. Wallace, Oxford University Press, 2002

Resources Available in Spanish

The Sjogren's Syndrome Foundation publishes a brochure on Sjogren's in Spanish. Contact the foundation for information at www.sjogrens.org, or call 800-475-6473. In addition, an information sheet on Sjogren's syndrome is available from the U.S. Department of Health and Human Services, National Institutes of Health, National Institute of Arthritis and Musculoskeletal and Skin Diseases.

See also *Síndrome de Sjogren,* by Juan-Manuel Anaya C., Manuel Ramos C., Mario Garcia C., Corpóracion Para Investigaciones Biológicas, Medellin,

Colombia, 2001, and (for professionals) *Síndrome de Sjogren*, edited by Manuel Ramos-Casals, Mario Barcia-Carrasco, Juan Manuel Anaya, Joaquim Coll, Ricard Cervera, Josep Font, Miguel Ingelmo, Masson, Barcelona, 2003

Textbooks in Rheumatology

Kelley's Textbook of Rheumatology, 6th edition, Shaun Ruddy et al. editors, Saunders, 2000

Arthritis and Allied Conditions: A Textbook of Rheumatology, 14th edition, William Koopman et al., Lippincott Williams and Wilkins, 2001

Clinical Primer of Rheumatology, William Koopman et al., editors, Lippincott Williams and Wilkins, 2003

Rheumatology, 3rd edition, Marc Hochberg et al., Mosby, 2003

Primer on the Rheumatic Diseases, John H. Klippel et al., editors, Arthritis Foundation, 2001

Treatment of the Rheumatic Diseases: A Companion to Kelley's Textbook of Rheumatology, Michael H. Weisman et al., Saunders, 2000

Oxford Textbook of Rheumatology, 2nd edition, P. J. Maddison et al., editors, Oxford University Press, 1998

Textbooks in Related Specialties

Burket's Oral Medicine: Diagnosis and Treatment, 10th edition, M. S. Greenberg and M Glick, editors, Decker, 2003

"Neurologic disease in Sjogren's syndrome," by Elaine Alexander, chapter 4 in *Systemic Diseases*, Part III, Handbook of Clinical Neurology vol. 27, no. 71, M. J. Aminoff and C. G. Goetz, editors, Elsevier Science, 1998

"Sjogren's Syndrome," by Ann L. Parke, chapter 57 in *Women and Health*, Marlene B. Goldman and Maureen C. Hatch, editors, Academic Press, 2000

Professional Societies

American College of Rheumatology (ACR): www.rheumatology.org

American Academy of Ophthalmology (AAO): www.aao.org

The Association for Research in Vision and Ophthalmology (ARVO): www .arvo.org

American Optometric Association (AOA): www.aoanet.org

American Dental Association (ADA): www.ada.org

International and American Associations of Dental Research (IADR/AADR): www.iadr.org

American Dental Education Association (ADEA): www.adea.org

American Dental Hygienists' Association (ADHA): www.adha.org

Bonnie T. Litton
Joan Manny
Katherine Morland Hammitt

Sjogren's Syndrome Foundation

APPENDIX 3
PRODUCTS FOR SJOGREN'S PATIENTS

Updates have been provided to the Sjogren's Syndrome Foundation for many years by many different people. The latest updates were compiled by Bonnie T. Litton, Joan Manny, and Katherine Morland Hammitt, who give special thanks to the many Sjogren's Syndrome Foundation members who contributed their suggestions that helped make this list possible. Sjogren's syndrome patients depend largely upon over-the-counter drugs and products to help ameliorate their symptoms, although some prescription drugs are now available for dry mouth and dry eye. Patients often need to try different products to see which ones work best for them and, especially in the case of prescription medications, have the least number of side effects. We do not attempt to list or discuss prescription medications for the systemic aspects of Sjogren's syndrome; these are covered in the relevant chapters, especially in Chapter 16, "Systemic Therapies in Sjogren's." Many patients want to know what products are available and which products have been tried and recommended by other patients. We must emphasize, however, that the list provided by the Sjogren's Syndrome Foundation can in no way be comprehensive. New products frequently come onto the market, and others are discontinued. Check with the foundation to obtain the latest list in booklet form or on the members-only section of the foundation Web site at www .sjogrens.org. We are also not acquainted with every product, so please contact the foundation if you, as a Sjogren's syndrome patient or health care professional who treats Sjogren's patients, find additional products that are especially helpful. The Sjogren's Syndrome Foundation in no way endorses any of the products mentioned in this listing. The products listed are those most frequently used by our members. We strongly advise that you check any medications, treatments, or products mentioned with your own physician, dentist, and/or pharmacist. Manufacturer phone numbers and Web site addresses are provided where available. Preservative-free products are indicated with an asterisk.

PRODUCTS FOR DRY EYE

Artificial Tears

The Sjogren's Syndrome Foundation's Medical and Scientific Advisory Board recommends that people who use artificial tears more than four times daily avoid products with preservatives. Consult your physician to see if you should use preservative-free products. If so, read labels carefully. Preservative-free products and those with preservatives often have similar sounding names. Preservatives often used in artificial tears include chlorobutanol, benzalkonium, and thimerosal.

Akwa Tears	800-535-7155	Akorn Inc. www.akorn.com
*Bion Tears	800-451-3937	Alcon Laboratories, Inc. www.alconlabs.com
Dakrina, Dwell (both by prescription)	800-969-6601	Apothecure Inc. www.apothecure.com
Healthy Relief Eye Drops #1	800-240-9780	Similasan Corporation www.healthyrelief.com
GenTeal Mild, GenTeal Moderate	888-669-6682	Novartis Ophthalmics www.novartisophthalmics .com
*GenTeal Lubricant Eye Drops—Single Dose	888-669-6682	Novartis Ophthalmics www.novartisophthalmics .com
*Moisture Eyes Lubricant Eye Drops/Artificial Tears	800-553-5340	Bausch & Lomb Pharmaceuticals, Inc. www.bausch.com
*Moisture Eyes Liquid Gel Lubricant Eye Drops	800-553-5340	Bausch & Lomb Pharmaceuticals, Inc. www.bausch.com
Murine Tears	877-854-0853	Prestige International Brands www.murine.com
Nature's Tears	800-272-5525	Watson Pharmaceuticals www.watsonpharm.com
*Nature's Tears EyeMist	800-367-6478	Rogue Springs Biologic Aqua Technologies www.naturestears.com

NutraTear	800-969-6601	Apothecure, Inc. www.apothecure.com
*Refresh Celluvisc	800-347-4500	Allergan, Inc. www.allergan.com
*Refresh Endura Lubricant Eye Drops	800-347-4500	Allergan, Inc. www.allergan.com
Refresh Liquigel Lubricant Eye Drops	800-347-4500	Allergan, Inc. www.allergan.com
*Refresh Tears and Refresh Plus	800-347-4500	Allergan, Inc. www.allergan.com
Rohto Zi for Eyes	800-688-7660	The Mentholatum Co. www.mentholatum.com
Sodium chloride solution 5%	800-535-7155	Akorn Inc. www.akorn.com
Systane	800-451-3937	Alcon Laboratories, Inc. www.alconlabs.com
Teargen, Teargen II	800-327-4114	IVAX Pharmaceuticals, Inc. www.ivaxpharmaceutical.com
*Tears Again Sterile Lubricant Liquid Gel	800-233-5469	Cynacon/OCuSOFT, Inc. www.ocusoft.com
*Tears Naturale Free	800-451-3937	Alcon Laboratories, Inc. www.alconlabs.com
Tears Renewed	800-535-7155	Akorn Inc. www.akorn.com
*TheraTears Liquid Gel Lubricant Eye Gel	800-579-8327	Advanced Vision Research www.theratears.com
*TheraTears Lubricant Eye Drops	800-579-8327	Advanced Vision Research www.theratears.com
*Viva Drops	800-325-6789	Vision Pharmaceuticals Inc. www.visionpharm.com

Artificial Tear Insert

*Lacrisert (prescription)	800-396-6250	Merck & Co. www.merck.com

Ocular Lubricants and Gels

Ocular lubricants are made with and without lanolin. You should consult with your physician to see if one or the other is better for you.

*AkwaTears Ointment	800-535-7155	Akorn Inc. www.akorn.com
GenTeal Lubricant Eye Gel— Severe	888-669-6682	Novartis Ophthalmics www.novartisophthalmics .com
Lacrilube Ointment	800-347-4500	Allergan, Inc. www.allergan.com
*Moisture Eyes PM Ointment	800-553-5340	Bausch & Lomb Pharma- ceuticals, Inc. www.bausch.com
*Puralube Ointment	800-645-9833	E. Fougera & Co. www.fougera.com
*Refresh PM Ointment	800-347-4500	Allergan, Inc. www.allergan.com
Sodium chloride 5% oph- thalmic ointment	800-535-7155	Akorn Inc. www.akorn.com
*Tears Again Night and Day Gel	800-233-5469	Cynacon/OCuSOFT, Inc. www.ocusoft.com
*Tears Naturale P.M. Lubricant Eye Ointment	800-451-3937	Alcon Laboratories, Inc. www.alconlabs.com
*Tears Renewed Ointment	800-535-7155	Akorn Inc. www.akorn.com

Additional Options for Dry Eye Relief

Tranquileyes Eye Hydrating Therapy	866-393-3267	Eyeeco www.eyeeco.com

Drugs That Decrease Inflammation and Increase Tear Flow

*Restasis (prescription)	800-347-4500	Allergan, Inc. www.allergan.com

Tablets/Capsules to Stimulate Lacrimal Gland Function

BioTears	888-303-2111	Biosyntrix, Inc. www.biosyntrix.com
Hydroeye	888-433-4726	Science Based Health www.sciencebasedhealth .com

Nutrition for the Eyes

Ocuvite Lutein	800-553-5340	Bausch & Lomb Pharma- ceuticals, Inc. www.bausch.com
TheraTears Nutrition for Dry Eyes	800-579-8327	Advanced Vision Research www.theratears.com

Tear Duct (Punctal) Plugs

Collagen Plugs (prescription) (collagen; dissolvable)	800-376-8327	Lacrimedics www.lacrimedics.com
Herrick Lacrimal Plug (prescription) (silicone; canalicular)	800-376-8327	Lacrimedics www.lacrimedics.com
Parasol Punctal Occluder System (temporary/removable)	888-905-7770	Odyssey Medical Inc. www.odysseymed.com
Punctum Plugs (prescription) (silicone; temporary/removable)	800-222-7584	Eagle Vision, Inc. www.eaglevis.com
Sharpoint (silicone; temporary/ removable)	800-523-3332	Surgical Specialties www.sharpoint.com
Smartplug (canalicular)	888-727-6100	Medennium Inc. www.medennium.com

Eye Wash Solutions

Bausch & Lomb Soothing Eye Wash	800-553-5340	Bausch & Lomb Pharmaceuticals, Inc. www.bausch.com
Collyrium for Fresh Eyes Eye Wash	800-553-5340	Bausch & Lomb Pharmaceuticals, Inc. www.bausch.com

Seasonal Allergy Conjunctivitis

Acular (prescription)	800-347-4500	Allergan, Inc. www.allergan.com

Vernal Conjunctivitis, Keratitis, and Keratoconjunctivitis

Alomide (prescription)	800-451-3937	Alcon Laboratories, Inc. www.alconlabs.com

Moisture Shields for the Eyes

Moist-Eye Moisture Panels	800-222-7584	Eagle Vision, Inc. www.eaglevis.com
Panoptx Windless Eyewear	877-726-6789	Panoptx www.panoptx.com
Wrap-Around Glasses	800-556-7170	Leonard Safety Equipment www.leonardsafety.com

Sterile Eyelid Cleansers

EyeScrub	866-451-5949	Novartis Ophthalmics www.novartisophthalmics .com
OCuSOFT Lid Scrub	800-233-5469	OCuSOFT, Inc. www.ocusoft.com

PRODUCTS FOR DRY MOUTH

Products That Stimulate Salivary Flow

Biotène Dry Mouth Gum	800-922-5856	Laclede, Inc. www.laclede.com
Evoxac (cevimeline HCl) (prescription)	877-324-4244	Daiichi Pharmaceutical Corp. www.daiichius.com
Salagen (pilocarpine) (prescription)	800-644-4811	MGI Pharma, Inc. www.mgipharma.com
Salix Saliva Stimulating Lozenges	800-288-2844	Scandinavian Natural Products www.scandinavian formulas.com
TheraGum with xylitol and calcium	800-643-3639	OMNII Oral Pharmaceuticals www.omniipharma.com
Xylichew Sugar Free Chewing Gum		Tundra Trading, Inc. www.tundratrading.com

Oral Moisturizers

Biotène Oral Balance Moisturizing Gel	800-922-5856	Laclede, Inc. www.laclede.com
Caphosol (prescription) (dispensed at compouding pharmacies)	781-864-2559	InPharma Inc. www.caphosol.com
Entertainer's Secret	800-308-7452	KLI Corp. www.entertainers-secret .com
Moi-Stir Solution and Moi-Stir Swabs	800-968-7772	Kingswood Labs, Inc. www.moi-stir.com
MouthKote with Yerba Santa	800-457-4276	Parnell Pharmaceuticals, Inc. www.parnellpharm.com

Orajel Dry Mouth Moisturizing Gel	800-952-5080	Del Laboratories www.orajel.com
Saliva Substitute	800-848-0120	Roxanne Laboratories, Inc. www.roxane.com
Salivart	800-321-9348	Gebauer Co. www.gebauerco.com
TheraSpray with xylitol	800-643-3639	OMNII Oral Pharmaceuticals www.omniipharma.com

Special Toothpastes, Mouthwashes, and Products and Devices for Cleaning Teeth

Aquafresh Toothpaste	888-825-5249	GlaxoSmithKline www.gsk.com
Biotène Antibacterial Dry Mouth Toothpaste Gentle Mint Gel Dry Mouth Toothpaste	800-922-5856	Laclede, Inc. www.laclede.com
Biotène Alcohol-Free Mouthwash	800-922-5856	Laclede, Inc. www.laclede.com
Colgate Total Floss	800-225-3756	Colgate Oral Pharmaceuticals www.colgateprofessional .com
ControlRx Toothpaste (prescription)	800-643-3639	OMNII Oral Pharmaceuticals www.omniipharma.com
FlossRx	800-643-3639	OMNII Oral Pharmaceuticals www.omniipharma.com
Glide Floss	800-645-4337	Procter & Gamble www.glidefloss.com
Orajel Dry Mouth Moisturizing Toothpaste	800-952-5080	Del Laboratories www.orajel.com
PerioMed	800-643-3639	OMNII Oral Pharmaceuticals www.omniipharma.com
Sensodyne Toothpaste	888-825-5249	GlaxoSmithKline www.gsk.com

| Sonicare—The Sonic Toothbrush | 800-682-7664 | Philips Oral Healthcare, Inc. www.sonicare.com |
| Squigle Enamel Saver Toothpaste | 877-718-0718 | Squigle, Inc. www.squigle.com |

Preparations to Protect and/or Remineralize Teeth

Caphosol (prescription) (dispensed at compounding pharmacies)	781-864-2559	Impharma Inc. www.caphosol.com
ControlRx Toothpaste (prescription) Neutral Sodium Fluoride	800-643-3639	OMNII Oral Pharmaceuticals www.omniipharma.com
Gel-Kam Gel (prescription) Stannous Fluoride	800-225-3756	Colgate Oral Pharmaceuticals www.colgateprofesional.com
Gel-Tin Liquid (prescription) Stannous Fluoride	800-325-1881	Young Dental Mfg. www.youngdental.com
OMNIIGel (prescription) Stannous Fluoride	800-643-3639	OMNII Oral Pharmaceuticals www.omniipharma.com
PreviDent Brush-on Sodium Fluoride Gel (prescription)	800-225-3756	Colgate Oral Pharmaceuticals www.colgateprofessional.com
PreviDent 5000 Plus (prescription) Sodium Fluoride	800-225-3756	Colgate Oral Pharmaceuticals www.colgateprofessional.com
Revive Gel	800-328-1276	Dental Resources Inc. www.dentalresourcesinc.com

Products to Soothe Dry Lips

Blistex Medicated Lip Ointment	888-784-2472	Blistex, Inc. www.blistex.com
Carmex Lip Moisturizer	414-421-7707	Carma Laboratories, Inc. www.carma-labs.com
Lip-Fix Cream	800-227-2445	Elizabeth Arden www.elizabetharden.com

Lip Medex	888-784-2472	Blistex, Inc. www.blistex.com
Neutrogena Lip Moisturizer	800-582-4048	Neutrogena Corp. www.neutrogena.com
Neutrogena Instant Lip Remedy, Neutrogena Over-night Lip Treatment	800-582-4048	Neutrogena Corp. www.neutrogena.com
Vaseline Lip Therapy	800-243-5804	Cheseborough-Ponds, Inc. www.unileverus.com

PRODUCTS FOR DRY NOSE

Moisturizers for Nasal Mucosal Tissue

Afrin Nasal Spray	908-298-4000	Schering-Plough Health-Care Products, Inc. www.schering-plough.com www.afrin.com
Ayr Saline Nasal Gel	800-324-1880	B.F. Ascher & Co., Inc. www.bfascher.com
Little Noses	800-754-8853	Little Remedies Products/ Vetco, Inc. www.littleremedies.com
Na-Zone	800-250-4258	Snuva, Inc. www.snuva.com
Ocean Nasal Spray	800-343-0164	Fleming & Co. www.flemingcompany.com
Pretz Spray with Yerba Santa	800-457-4276	Parnell Pharmaceuticals, Inc. www.parnellpharm.com
Sinus Rinse	877-477-8633	NeilMed Products, Inc. www.nasalrinse.com

PRODUCTS FOR DRY SKIN

Moisturizers, Creams, and Cleansing Products

| AmLactin Cream and Lotion | 800-654-2299 | Upsher-Smith
www.upsher-smith.com |
| Aveeno moisturizing lotions and cream | 877-298-2525 | Johnson & Johnson Consumer Products
www.aveeno.com |

Bag Balm	800-232-3610	Dairy Association Co, Inc. www.bagbalm.com
Borage Therapy Body Lotion and Hand Cream	800-448-0298	ShiKai Products www.shikai.com
Carmol 20	800-929-9300	Bradley Pharmaceuticals, Inc. www.bradpharm.com
Cetaphil moisturizing lotions		Galderma Laboratories, L.P. www.cetaphil.com
Curel Ultra Healing Therapy Lotion	800-572-2931	The Andrew Jergens Company www.curel.com
Derm-Apply Moisturizing Lotion	800-250-4258	Snuva, Inc. www.snuva.com
Eucerin Moisturizing Lotion and Eucerin Dry Skin Therapy	800-227-4703	Beiersdof Inc. www.eucerinus.com
Glycerin Hand Therapy	800-541-8647	Camille Beckman www.camillebeckman online.com
Lac-Hydrin (prescription)		Bristol Meyers Squibb www.bms.com
Lubriderm for Sensitive Skin and Lubriderm Skin Therapy	800-223-0182	Pfizer Consumer Healthcare www.prodhelp.com
Neutrogena Norwegian Formula Body Cream, and Hand Cream	800-582-4048	Neutrogena Corp. www.neutrogena.com
Nivea Extra Enriched Lotions	800-227-4703	Beiersdorf Inc. www.niveausa.com
St. Ives with Vitamin E and Advanced Therapy Lotion, St. Ives Intensive Healing		St. Ives Laboratories, Inc. www.stives.com/products
Vanicream Skin Cream and Vanicream Lite Lotion	800-325-8232	Pharmaceutical Specialties, Inc. www.vanicream.com
Vitec Vitamin E Lotion	800-325-8232	Pharmaceutical Specialties, Inc. www.paico.com

| Zim's Crack Creme | 800-319-2225 | Perfecta Products www.crackcreme.com |

Other commonly used products that patients listed and that should be easy to find at your local drug store include Basis Soap, Keri Lotion, Johnson's Baby Oil with aloe vera and Vitamin E, Moisturel, and Vaseline Water Resistant Lotion.

PRODUCTS FOR VAGINAL DRYNESS

Astroglide, Silken Secret	800-848-5900	BioFilm, Inc. www.astroglide.com
Estrace Vaginal Cream (prescription)	800-521-8813	Warner Chilcottt www.warnerchilcott.com
Feminease	800-457-4276	Parnell Pharmaceuticals, Inc. www.parnellpharm.com
K-Y Long Lasting Vaginal Moisturizer	877-592-7263	Personal Products Co.
Lubrin Vaginal Inserts	973-882-1505	Bradley Pharmaceuticals, Inc. www.bradpharm.com
Maxilube Personal Lubricant	800-531-3333	Mission Pharmacal Co. www.missionpharmacal.com
Premarin Vaginal Cream (prescription)	800-934-5556	Wyeth Pharmaceuticals www.wyeth.com
Replens Long-Lasting Vaginal Moisturizer	877-507-6516	LDS Consumer Products www.replens.com

HUMIDIFIERS

| Kaz Personal Humidifier | 800-827-6712 | KAZ Home Environment www.kaz.com |
| Venta Airwasher | 888-333-8218 | Venta-Airwasher LLC www.venta-airwasher.com |

FOOTWEAR FOR NEUROPATHY PAIN

| Thor-Lo Walking Crew WX-11 S | 888-846-7567 | THOR-LO, Inc. www.thorlo.com |

PRODUCTS AND MEDICATIONS FOR REFLUX

Antacids are often the first line of defense against reflux and include those that contain aluminum and magnesium salts (for example, Alka-Seltzer, Maalox, Mylanta, Pepto-Bismol, Rolaids, and Riopan) and those that contain calcium carbonate (for example, Tums, Titralac, and Alka-2). Foaming agents such as Gaviscon, to help combat reflux, can also be found over the counter.

H2 Blockers

H2 blockers are available over the counter or in greater strengths by prescription.

Axid AR (nizatidine)	800-545-5979	Eli Lilly and Company Limited www.lilly.com
Pepcid AC (famotidine)	800-755-4008	Merck Consumer Pharmaceuticals Co. www.pepcidac.com
Tagamet HB (cimetidine)	800-482-4394	GlaxoSmithKline www.tagamethb.com
Zantac 75 (ranitidine)	888-825-5249	GlaxoSmithKline www.gsk.com

Proton Pump Inhibitors

Aciphex (rabeprazole) (prescription)		Janssen Pharmaceutica Inc. www.aciphex.com
Nexium (esomeprazole) (prescription)	800-236-9933	AstraZeneca LP www.purplepill.com
Prevacid (iansoprazole) (prescription)	800-621-1020	TAP Pharmaceutical Products Inc. www.prevacid.com
Prilosec (omeprazole)	800-236-9933	AstraZeneca LP www.priloseconline.com
Protonix (pantoprazole) (prescription)	800-934-5556	Wyeth Pharmaceuticals www.protonixrx.com

APPENDIX 4
GLOSSARY

achlorhydria: Gastric acid deficiency.

ACR (American College of Rheumatology): A professional association of United States rheumatologists. Criteria (definitions) of many rheumatic diseases are called the *ACR Criteria*.

adenopathy: A swelling of the lymph nodes. In Sjogren's syndrome, this usually occurs in the neck and jaw region.

alopecia: Hair loss.

albumin: A protein that circulates in the blood and carries materials to cells.

alveoli: Air sacs of the lungs.

amylase: An enzyme present in saliva; another form of amylase is produced by the pancreas.

Analgesic: A drug that alleviates pain.

angular cheilitis: Sores at the corners of the mouth (angles of the lips).

antibody: Substance in the blood that is normally made in response to infection. Also referred to as immunoglobulins such as IgG, IgM, etc.

anticentromere antibody: Antibodies to a cell nucleus associated with scleroderma.

anticardiolipin antibody: An antiphospholipid antibody.

anti-DNA (anti-double-stranded DNA): Antibodies to DNA; seen in half of patients with lupus.

anti-ENA (extractable nuclear antibodies): A group of antibodies that includes anti-Sm and anti-RNP.

antigen(s): A chemical substance that provokes the production of antibody. In tetanus vaccination, for example, tetanus is the antigen injected to produce antibodies and hence protective immunity to tetanus.

antimalarial drugs: Quinine-derived drugs, which were first developed to treat malaria and can manage Sjogren's, such as hydroxychloroquine (Plaquenil).

antinuclear antibodies (ANA): Autoantibodies directed against components in the nucleus of the cell. Screening test for lupus and other connective tissue diseases including Sjogren's syndrome.

antispasmodic drugs: Medications that quiet spasms. Usually used in reference to the gastrointestinal tract.

antiphospholipid antibody: Antibodies to a constituent of cell membranes seen in one-third of those with SLE. In the presence of a cofactor, these antibodies can alter clotting and lead to strokes, blood clots, miscarriages, and low platelet counts. Also detected as the lupus anticoagulant.

anti-RNP: Antibody to ribonucleoprotein. Seen in lupus and mixed connective tissue disease.

anti-Sm: Anti-Smith antibody; found only in lupus.

anti-SSA (Ro antibody): Associated with Sjogren's syndrome, sun sensitivity, neonatal lupus, and congenital heart block.

anti-SSB (La antibody): Almost always seen with anti-SSA.

apoptosis: Programmed cell death.

arteriole: A very small artery.

arthralgia: Pain in a joint.

arthritis: Inflammation of a joint.

ascites: An abnormal fluid that collects in the abdomen due to certain liver and other disorders.

atrophy: A thinning of the surface; a form of wasting.

autoantibody: Antibody that attacks the body's own tissues and organs as if they were foreign.

autoimmunity: A state in which the body inappropriately produces antibody against its own tissues. The antigens are components of the body.

B cell or B lymphocyte: A white blood cell that makes antibodies.

basal (resting) rate: Unstimulated (used in reference to both tears and salivary flow).

bolus: A morsel of food, already chewed, ready to be swallowed.

bronchi: Branches of the trachea.

buffer: A mixture of acid or base that, when added to a solution, enables the solution to resist changes in the pH that would otherwise occur when acid or alkali is added to it.

cartilage: Tissue material covering bone. The nose, outer ears, and trachea consist primarily of cartilage.

chronic active hepatitis: A disorder that occurs when viral hepatitis proceeds in an active state beyond its usual cause.

calcification: A process in which tissue or noncellular material in the body becomes hardened as the result of deposits of insoluble calcium salts.

candidiasis: Moniliasis. A condition due to an overgrowth of the yeast (fungus) candida.

cariostatic: Having the ability to help prevent dental caries.

celiac disease: Gluten intolerance.

complete blood count (CBC): A blood test measuring the amount of red cells, white blood cells, and platelets in the body.

congenital heart block: A dysfunction of the rate/rhythm conduction system in the fetal or infant heart.

central nervous system: The brain and spinal cord.

collagen vascular disease: *See* connective tissue disease.

connective tissue disease: A disorder marked by inflammation of the connective tissue (joints, skin, muscles) in multiple areas. In most instances, connective tissue diseases are associated with autoimmunity.

cornea: The clear "watch crystal" structure covering the pupil and iris (colored portion of the eye). It is composed of several vital layers, all of which are functionally important. The surface layer, or epithelium, is covered by the tears, which lubricate and protect the surface.

corticosteroid: A hormone produced by the adrenal cortex gland. Natural adrenal gland hormones have powerful anti-inflammatory activity and are often used in the treatment of severe inflammation affecting vital organs. The many side effects of corticosteroids should markedly curtail their use in mild disorders.

crossover syndrome: An autoimmune process that has features of more than one rheumatic disease.

cryoglobulins: Protein complexes circulating in the blood that are precipitated during cold.

cryptogenic cirrhosis: Liver disease of unknown etiology (origin) in patients with no history of alcoholism or previous acute hepatitis.

dermatomyositis: An autoimmune process directed against muscles associated with skin rashes.

diuretics: Medications that increase the body's ability to rid itself of fluids.

double-blind study: One in which neither the physician nor the patients being treated know whether patients are receiving the active ingredient being tested or a placebo (an inactive substance).

dysorexia: Impaired or deranged appetite.

dysphagia: Difficulty in swallowing. In Sjogren's syndrome this may be attributable to several causes, among them a decrease in saliva, infiltration of the glands at the esophageal mucosa, or esophageal webbing.

dyspnea: Air hunger resulting in labored or difficult breathing, sometimes accompanied by pain.

ecchymosis: A purplish patch caused by oozing of blood into the skin; ecchymoses differ from petechiae in size.

edema: Swelling caused by retention of fluid.

ELISA (enzyme-linked immunosorbent assay): A very sensitive blood test for detecting the presence of autoantibodies.

epistaxis: Nosebleed or hemorrhaging from the nose, which may be caused by dryness of the nasal mucous membrane in Sjogren's syndrome.

erythema: A medical term for a red color, usually associated with increased blood flow to an inflamed area, often the skin.

erythrocyte: Red blood cell.

esophagus: A canal (narrow tube) with muscular walls allowing passage of food from the pharynx, or end of the mouth, to the stomach.

erythrocyte sedimentation rate (ESR): Measures the speed at which a column of blood settles. Most common and simple test for inflammation.

etiology: The cause(s) of a disease.

eustachian tube: The tube running from the back of the nose to the middle ear.

exocrine glands: Glands that secrete mucus.

exocrinopathy: Disease related to the exocrine glands.

exocrine glands: A gland that secretes outwardly through ducts.

fibromyalgia: A form of non-neuropathic chronic neuromuscular pain associated with fatigue, disordered sleeping, and tender points in the soft tissues.

fibrosis: Abnormal formation of fibrous tissue.

fissure: A crack in the tissue surface (skin, tongue, etc.).

fluorescein stain: A dye that stains areas of the eye surface in which cells have been lost.

gastritis: Stomach inflammation.

gene: Consisting of DNA, it is the basic unit of inherited information in our cells.

genetic factors: Traits inherited from parents, grandparents, and so on.

gingiva: The gums.

gingivitis: Inflammation of the gums.

granuloma: A nodular, inflammatory lesion.

human leukocyte antigens (HLA): A group of genes that governs the ability of lymphocytes, such as T cells and B cells, to respond to foreign and self substances.

idiopathic: Of unknown cause.

immunogenetics: The study of genetic factors that control the immune response.

immunoglobulin E (IgE): Antibody associated with allergies.

immunoglobulins (gamma globulins): The protein fraction of serum responsible for antibody activity. Measurement of serum immunoglobulin levels can serve as a guide to disease activity in some patients with Sjogren's syndrome.

immunomodulators: Medications that affect the body's immune system.

immunosuppressive agents: A class of drugs that interferes with the function of cells composing the immune system. *See* lymphocyte.

immunosuppressive agents. Drugs used in the chemotherapy of malignant disease and in the prevention of transplant rejection are generally immunosuppressive and occasionally are used to treat severe autoimmune disease.

incisal: Cutting edge (of a tooth).

interstitial: Supporting structure of the substance of an organ or tissues.

interstitial nephritis: Inflammation of the connective tissue of the kidney, usually resulting in mild kidney disease characterized by frequent urination. Interstitial nephritis may be associated with Sjogren's syndrome.

intraoral: Inside the mouth.

keratoconjunctivitis sicca: Condition, also called dry eye, that most frequently occurs in women in their forties and fifties. If it is associated with a dry mouth and/or rheumatoid arthritis, the condition is referred to as Sjogren's syndrome.

lacrimal: Relating to the tears.

lacrimal glands: Two types of glands that produce tears. Smaller accessory glands in the eyelid tissue produce the tears needed from minute to minute. The main lacrimal glands, located just inside the bony tissue surrounding the eye, produce large amounts of tears.

larynx: Voice box.

latent: Not manifest but potentially discernible.

lip biopsy: Incision of approximately 2 cm on the inside surface of the lower lip and excision of some of the minor salivary glands for microscopic examination and analysis.

lymph: A fluid collected from the tissues throughout the body, flowing through the lymph nodes and eventually added to the circulating blood.

lymphocyte: A type of white blood cell concerned with antibody production and regulation. Collections of lymphocytes are seen in the salivary glands of Sjogren's syndrome patients.

lymphoma: A severe proliferation (increase) of abnormal (malignant) lymphocytes, manifested as cancer of the lymph glands. Although exceedingly rare, lymphoma occurring as a complication of severe Sjogren's syndrome has been identified by immunologists.

matrix: The section of the tooth enamel that holds calcium and phosphate minerals.

mixed connective tissue disease: A connective tissue disease that manifests as an overlap of other connective-tissue disorders.

Meibomian glands: Fat-producing glands in the eyelids that produce an essential component of tears.

mucin: Thinnest layer of the tear film; layer closest to the cornea.

mucolytic agents: Medications that tend to dissolve mucus. Most patients with dry eye complain of excess mucous discharge. Some patients may benefit from these medications if other tear-film-enhancing drops are not very effective.

necrosis: Tissue death.

nephritis: An inflammation of the kidneys.

neutrophil: A granulated white blood cell involved in bacterial killing and acute inflammation.

nonspecific: Caused by other diseases or multiple factors.

nonsteroidal anti-inflammatory drugs (NSAIDS): Anti-inflammatory agents blocking the action of prostaglandins used to treat pain that occur in rheumatoid arthritis and other connective-tissue disorders. Examples include ibuprofen (Motrin, Advil) and naproxen (Aleve).

olfactory: Relating to the sense of smell.

ophthalmologist: A physician who specializes in diseases and surgery of the eye.

oral mucosa: The lining (mucous membrane) of the mouth.

oral soft tissue: Tongue, mucous lining of the cheeks, and lips.

otitis: Inflammation of the ear, which may be marked by pain, fever, abnormalities of hearing, deafness, tinnitus (a ringing sensation), and vertigo. In Sjogren's syndrome, blockage at eustachian tubes due to infection can lead to conduction deafness and chronic otitis.

otolaryngologist: Physician specializing in ear, nose, and throat disorders.

palate biopsy: A punch biopsy near the junction of the hard and soft palates to sample the minor salivary glands in that region.

palpable: Perceptible to touch.

parasympathetic nervous system: The part of the autonomic nervous system whose functions include constriction of the pupils of the eyes, slowing of the heartbeat, and stimulation of certain digestive glands. These nerves originate in the midbrain, the hindbrain, and the sacral region of the spinal cord; impulses are mediated by acetylcholine.

parotid gland flow: An empirical quantitative measure of the amount of saliva produced over a certain period of time. Normal parotid gland flow rate is 1.5 ml/min. In Sjogren's syndrome, the flow rate is approximately 0.5 ml/min, with diminution of the flow rate correlating inversely with the severity of disease.

parotid glands: One of the three pairs of major salivary glands. They are located in front of the ear.

pericardium: The lining of the heart.

photosensitivity: Sensitivity to ultraviolet light.

pleura: A sac lining the lung.

primary biliary cirrhosis (PBC): Impairment of bile excretion secondary to liver inflammation and scarring.

perforation: A hole.

pericarditis: Inflammation of the lining of the heart.

periodontitis: Inflammation of the tissues surrounding and supporting the teeth.

peripheral nerves: Nerves outside the central nervous system.

petechia: A small, pinpoint, nonraised, perfectly round, purplish red spot caused by intradermal or submucosal hemorrhaging.

pharynx: Throat.

placebo: An inactive substance used as a "dummy" medication.

plaque: A thin, sticky film that builds up on the teeth, trapping harmful bacteria.

plasma: The fluid portion of the circulating blood.

pleurisy: Inflammation of the pleura (membrane surrounding the lungs and lining the walls of the rib cavity).

polymyositis: A connective tissue disorder characterized by muscle pain and severe weakness secondary to inflammation in the major voluntary muscles.

psoralen: A drug administered orally or topically for the treatment of vitiligo (white patches caused by loss of pigment).

puncta: Small holes in the eyelids that normally drain tears. Patients with severe dry eye benefit from punctal closure, which allows maximal tear preservation.

purpura: A condition characterized by hemorrhage into the skin, appearing as crops of petechiae (very small red spots).

radioactive isotope: Radioactive material used in diagnostic tests.

radionuclide studies: A technique in which radioactive isotopes, such as radiolabeled human serum albumin, are injected into an organ. A gamma scintillation camera, coupled with a digital computer system and a cathode ray display, reads the radioactive emissions. Areas of perfusion will show marked radiographic emissions; areas of obstruction will show no activity.

Raynaud's phenomenon: Painful blanching of the fingertips on exposure to cold. This may be seen alone or in association with a connective tissue disease.

reflux: A regurgitation due to the return of gas, fluid, or small amount of food from the stomach.

renal: Relating to the kidneys.

rheumatoid arthritis: A form of arthritis characterized by inflammation of the joints, stiffness, swelling, synovial hypertrophy, and pain.

rheumatoid factor: An autoantibody whose presence in the blood usually indicates autoimmune activity.

rheumatologist: A physician skilled in the diagnosis and treatment of rheumatic conditions.

rose bengal: A dye that stains abnormal or sick cells on the surface of the eye. This diagnostic dye allows the ophthalmologist to follow the treatment of dry eye.

salicylates: Aspirin-like drugs.

salivary scintigraphy: Measurement of salivary gland function through injection of radioactive material.

sarcoidosis: A systemic disease with granulomatous (nodular, inflammatory) lesions involving the lungs and, on occasion, the salivary glands, with resulting fibrosis.

Schirmer test: The standard objective test to diagnose dry eye. Small pieces of filter paper are placed between the lower eyelid and eyeball and soak up the tears for five minutes. The value obtained is a rough estimation of tear production in relative terms. Lower values are consistent with dry eye. It is important to emphasize that no single test can be considered diagnostic unless the condition is severe.

scleroderma: A connective tissue disorder characterized by thickening and hardening of the skin. Sometimes internal organs (intestines, kidneys) are affected, causing bowel irregularity and high blood pressure.

secretogogue: A medication that can stimulate salivary flow.

serum: The fluid portion of the blood (obtained after removal of the fibrin clot and blood cells), distinguished from the plasma in the circulation blood.

sialochemistry: Measurement of the constituents in saliva.

sialography: X-ray examination of the salivary duct system by use of liquid contrast medium. Radiologically sensitive dye is placed into the duct system, outlining the system clearly.

signs: Changes that can be seen or measured.

Sjogren's antibodies: Abnormal antibodies found in the sera of Sjogren's syndrome patients. These antibodies react with the extracts of certain cells, and a test based on this principle can be helpful in the diagnosis of Sjogren's syndrome. *See also* SSA and SSB.

Sjogren's syndrome: A symptom complex of dry eye, dry mouth, and dryness of other mucous membranes associated with inflammation of the lacrimal and/or salivary glands. It can occur alone (50 percent) or in association with a connective tissue disease.

SLE (systemic lupus erythematosus): An inflammatory connective tissue disease.

SSA: Sjogren's syndrome–associated antigen A (anti-Ro).

SSB: Sjogren's syndrome–associated antigen B (anti-La).

steatorrhea: Passage of large amounts of fat in the feces, as occurs in pancreatic disease and the malabsorption syndromes.

steroids: Cortisone-derived medications.

sublingual glands: One of the three pairs of major salivary glands. They are located in the floor of the mouth under the tongue.

submandibular glands: One of the three pairs of major salivary glands. They are located below the lower jaw.

symptoms: Changes patients feel.

systemic: Any process that involves multiple organ systems throughout the body.

synovitis: Inflammation of the tissues lining a joint.

synovium: Tissue that lines a joint.

T cell: A lymphocyte (white blood cell) responsible for immunologic memory.

thymus: A gland in the neck responsible for immunologic memory.

thrush: A form of candidiasis. Infection of the oral tissues with *Candida albicans*.

thyroiditis: A disease in which autoantibodies cause immune system cells (lymphocytes) to destroy the thyroid gland.

titer: Test showing the strength or concentration of a particular volume of a solution. Usually refers to amounts of antibody present.

TMJ (temporomandibular joint): The joint of the lower jaw where the ball-and-socket arrangement is formed by the condyle of the lower jaw (the ball) and the fossa of the temporal bone (the socket). The joint space is filled with synovial or lubricating fluid. This joint and the surrounding synovial tissues may become inflamed if rheumatoid arthritis accompanies Sjogren's syndrome and involves the joint.

trachea: Windpipe.

tracheobronchial tree: The windpipe and the bronchi into which it subdivides.

UCTD (undifferentiated connective tissue disease): Features of autoimmunity such as inflammatory arthritis or Raynaud's in a patient who does not meet the ACR criteria for lupus, rheumatoid arthritis or other disorders.

ultraviolet light (UV light): A spectrum of light including UVA (320–400 nanometers), UVB (290–320 nanometers), and UVC (200–290 wavelengths).

urticaria: Hives.

vasculitis: Inflammation of a blood vessel.

venule: A very small vein.

viscera: The organs of the digestive, respiratory, urogenital, and endocrine systems, as well as the spleen, heart, and great vessels (blood and lymph ducts).

vitiligo: White patches on the skin due to loss of pigment.

xerophthalmia: Dry eyes.

xerostomia: Dryness of the mouth caused by the arresting of normal salivary secretions. It occurs in diabetes, drug therapy, radiation therapy, and Sjogren's syndrome.

xylitol: A sweetening agent with cariostatic properties.

INDEX

ACE (angiotensin-converting enzyme) inhibitors, 88
acid reflux (gastro-esophageal reflux), 38, 73, 79, 88, 136, 142, 249
acinar cells, 18, 58
acupuncture, 126, 182, 185
acute phase reactants, 98–99
adenopathy (lymph node swelling), 12, 21, 92, 111
age of onset, 11, 12, 82, 108
aging, comorbidity of, 201–2
AIDS. *See* HIV
alcohol, 148, 150, 153
allergic conjunctivitis, 50
allergies, 107, 194
allopurinol, 132
alternative medicine. *See* complementary and alternative medicine (CAM)
ambroxol, 130–31
American College of Rheumatology (ACR), 84, 95, 194
American-European Consensus Group, 186
amiloride (diuretic), 133, 134, 142
amylase (enzyme), 74
androgens, 19
anemia, 74, 79, 137, 141, 142
anetholetrithione, 127
anger, coping with, 160–62, 168
angular cheilitis, 63
anti-acetylcholine muscarinic receptors, 102
antiallergy medications, 44, 50
anti-alpha-fodrin (autoantibody), 102–3
antibodies, 46, 58, 61; anticardiolipin, 198–99; antimitochondrial, 75, 137; antineurophil cytoplasmic (ANCA), 91; antiphospholipid, 85, 86–87, 198–99; and congenital heart block, 76–77. *See also* antinuclear antibodies (ANAs); autoantibodies
antidepressants, 45, 107, 164
antidiuretic hormone (ADH), 133–34
anti-DNA (anti-double-stranded DNA), 85
antihistamines, 32, 107

anti-inflammatory medications, 180, 181. *See also* NSAIDs
anti-La/SSB antibody, 4, 7, 27, 29, 93, 195–98; and congenital heart block, 76–77, 196–98; tests for, 85, 94, 97, 101–2
antimalarial drugs, 86, 140–41, 143
antimitochondrial antibodies (AMAs), 75, 137
anti-muscarinic receptor, 28
antineurophil cytoplasmic antibodies (ANCA), 91
antinuclear antibodies (ANA), 12, 27–28, 84, 85, 90; test for, 94, 97, 100
antiphospholipid antibody syndrome (APS), 86–87, 198–200
anti-Ro/SSA antibody, 4, 7, 11, 27, 29, 195–98; and congenital heart block, 76–77, 196–98; testing for, 12, 85, 94, 97, 101–2, 187
apoptosis (cell death), 20
arthritis, 37–38; osteoarthritis, 146, 178, 180, 181, 182, 184. *See also* rheumatoid arthritis
Arthritis Foundation, 170
artificial saliva, 123
artificial tear preparations, 116, 117–18, 239–40
atrophic gastritis, 73–74, 137
atrophic rhinitis, 54
autoantibodies, 25–29, 31, 35, 90, 195–96; sicca symptoms, 81; testing for, 102–3
autoimmune disease, xv, 7, 11, 12, 95; causes of, 220; testing for, 97, 110–12; theories of, 18, 20–23; women and, 19. *See also specific condition*
Autoimmune Diseases Research Plan, 220
autonomic nervous system, 38
Ayurvedic medicine, 182–83
azathioprine, 70, 75, 90, 132, 144

bacteria: and saliva, 17, 61; and tooth decay, 61, 62, 123

259